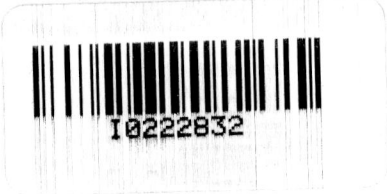

FAT IN FOUR CULTURES

Fat in Four Cultures

A Global Ethnography of Weight

CINDI STURTZSREETHARAN

ALEXANDRA BREWIS

JESSICA HARDIN

SARAH TRAINER

AMBER WUTICH

TC⊳ TEACHING CULTURE

UNIVERSITY OF TORONTO PRESS
Toronto Buffalo London

© University of Toronto Press 2021
Toronto Buffalo London
utorontopress.com

ISBN 978-1-4875-0800-5 (cloth)   ISBN 978-1-4875-3736-4 (EPUB)
ISBN 978-1-4875-2562-0 (paper)   ISBN 978-1-4875-3735-7 (PDF)

Library and Archives Canada Cataloguing in Publication

Title: Fat in four cultures : a global ethnography of weight / Cindi SturtzSreetharan, Alexandra Brewis, Jessica Hardin, Sarah Trainer, Amber Wutich.
Names: SturtzSreetharan, Cindi, author. | Brewis, Alexandra, author. | Hardin, Jessica A., author. | Trainer, Sarah, author. | Wutich, Amber, author.
Series: Teaching culture.
Description: Series statement: Teaching culture : UTP ethnographies for the classroom | Includes bibliographical references and index.
Identifiers: Canadiana (print) 20210153962 | Canadiana (ebook) 20210154160 | ISBN 9781487525620 (paper) | ISBN 9781487508005 (cloth) | ISBN 9781487537364 (EPUB) | ISBN 9781487537357 (PDF)
Subjects: LCSH: Obesity – Cross-cultural studies. | LCSH: Body image – Cross-cultural studies. | LCSH: Stigma (Social psychology) – Cross-cultural studies.
Classification: LCC RA645.O23 S78 2021 | DDC 362.1963/98–dc23

We welcome comments and suggestions regarding any aspect of our publications – please feel free to contact us at news@utorontopress.com or visit us at utorontopress .com.

Every effort has been made to contact copyright holders; in the event of an error or omission, please notify the publisher.

University of Toronto Press acknowledges the financial assistance to its publishing program of the Canada Council for the Arts and the Ontario Arts Council, an agency of the Government of Ontario.

Canada Council   Conseil des Arts
for the Arts   du Canada

ONTARIO ARTS COUNCIL
CONSEIL DES ARTS DE L'ONTARIO
an Ontario government agency
un organisme du gouvernement de l'Ontario

Funded by the   Financé par le
Government   gouvernement
of Canada   du Canada

Canadä

Contents

Foreword

Fat is a powerful symbol. Wealth, poverty, conviviality, shame, youth, age, power, weakness. These symbols have all been associated with fat and are deeply rooted in historical and cultural knowledge, which shifts with time. Fat is not the same everywhere. Yet its symbolism travels. It sits within silences and spaces of exchange, of words, foods, ideas, and currencies. It also can be seen, interpreted, and communicated in various ways across borders, as well as disciplines.

Children travel with ideas about their bodies and society throughout life. Mimi Nichter exemplified this in her book, *Fat Talk,* when she spoke of Wendy, a curly-haired, heavy-set freshman in Tuscon, Arizona, who was trying to lose forty pounds and "was acutely aware of weight-related stereotypes even though she had a supportive group of friends."[1] This book similarly travels. As anthropologists, we carry our ways of thinking and being in the world to field sites in which we work, which may require minutes, hours, or days of travel to reach. The anthropologists who collaborated in the writing of this book have worked around the world in more projects that I can count. They bring together decades of thinking, learning, observing, and seeking to interpret how fat travels: through time, space, between the ears (cognitive), and between the noses (interactive).

Fat is inherently a social category that causes varied emotions and responses from place to place. I remember how my host mom called me *gordita* (translated, chubby girl) when I returned to Valparaíso after spending six weeks learning, listening, and interviewing women in a clinic in Carahue, Chile, during my junior year of university study abroad. I blushed and smiled, while my mind was racing because I had definitely gained weight as I ate all the delicious food my host mom in Carahue prepared. I also had had no time to exercise, as I usually would to release anxiety and find balance. Later that day, I laced up my sneakers and headed out for a run. I have never been typically thin, but I remember the anxiety this comment caused me, as I was enculturated into a society that believes "having a good body is a form of control and a source of empowerment because it opens up more choices in life."[2] But my host mom meant to compliment me – while my Euro-American upbringing interpreted it as criticism (even while knowing what it was *supposed* to mean).

Talking about people's bodies can be hard. I have interviewed hundreds of people, mostly women, around the world whose bodies may or may not align with their idealized vision of beauty. Many people I work with have been diagnosed with diabetes (often type 2), and many have thicker middles. But people don't think about it the same way everywhere, and definitely not everyone who gets diabetes later in life would define themselves as fat. But many people describe their bodies – the shapes, feelings, changes – temporally, as they reflect on periods of their lives. I have found that trauma and change can be inscribed in the body and relational to how women perceive their journey. This is not the same everywhere, but consistent everywhere I have worked.[3]

Most of my work involves teams. However, in my case, I have traveled to join existing teams who worked before and after my arrival together on similar questions. What I did was dig deeper into social, cultural, and phenomenological experiences, while my colleagues often worked with bigger datasets, which in most cases were biologically oriented or clinically facing. This type of work departs from a view of anthropology as a solo endeavor – something that I have never found to be real. In my experience, everything is collaborative in some way, and recognizing how we generate ideas with others is critical. This book provides another model for generating cross-cultural thinking of how people think and live in their bodies.

The authors of this book reveal a powerful story, weaving together ethnographic moments with collective design, analysis, and writing. I cannot hide my jealousy of the time they spent talking together about ideas, ethnography, mothering, writing, reflexivity, and collective knowledge. This book provides not only the most nuanced cross-cultural analysis of fat and culture to date but also sets the stage for a shift in medical anthropology toward more collective ethnographic and comparative work.

I remember sitting in the audience of a talk in the mid-2000s at the American Anthropological Association Annual Meeting when Jennifer Hirsch and her colleagues presented preliminary work that culminated in *The Secret*.[4] I left with my head chock full of new ideas and I was filled with excitement about what cross-cultural, collaborative ethnographic work might look like. This book paved the way for culturally grounded comparisons in anthropology that speak to public health and can move well beyond anthropological silos. *Fat in Four Cultures* shares this reflexive knowledge that speaking within and between disciplinary landscapes can move the needle on how people talk about fat. But, more than that, it speaks to the power of culture and symbols that define who we are and how we collectively cherish one another.

This book also shines a light on the power and rigor of ethnographic methods. The anthropologists writing this book have set a high bar for defining how collaborative methods work, and how cross-cultural ethnography can be systematic and transparent. Indeed, some might argue that this kind of transparency of anthropological methods is a radical act – something anthropologists are known to have pushed against for decades. They lift the lid on the words people use, what those words mean and are supposed to mean, and how people internalize or externalize the meaning of fat in their lives and society at large. In doing so, they exemplify the power of ethnographic writing and the complexity of collective analysis.

I would be remiss if I did not mention the relevance and power of this book following and speaking to, or beyond, *Birth in Four Cultures*.[5] I will admit that I did not read this book until I had completed my doctoral studies and was pregnant with my first child. I conceived in South Africa and received four months of prenatal care there; then I received follow-up care in the United States while I hid my pregnancy and interviewed for jobs. I spent the second half of my pregnancy in England and delivered at the Whittington Hospital, four blocks from where my great-grandmother spent the last four decades of her life. Working through the meaning of my body, change, pregnancy, being far from my mother and sister, and justifying what we were doing bringing a child into the world amidst extraordinary personal and global precarity brought me to read *Birth in Four Cultures* (and admittedly, many more books about birth, fear, love, and motherhood). I found this book drove home the fact that we cannot expect universality or complete relativism, and that I need to think and move within multiple paradigms and systems. In the introduction to the fourth edition, the authors highlight that, "while we find a low level of variation *within* any given system, the range of variation in specific practices *across* different systems is expectably extensive."[6] Even so, I planned for a completely natural birth and had the most medicated one I could have expected. In this way, our perceptions and beliefs do not always relate to our experience – something anthropologists are particularly skilled at drawing out in their fieldwork. *Fat in Four Cultures* similarly demonstrates the cultural relativity of fat, while going to great extent to explain and deconstruct how variation within contexts is a powerful and personal experience.

My youngest daughter just walked into the room, minutes before my writing time for the day expires. She sang a song for me as she showed me a map of the world she made in her Montessori school. She said, "I made all the continents!" Similarly, this book provides a walk through the continents and a deep dive into how people experience not only how the world is changing but also what people interpret the inscriptions of this world on our bodies to mean. The symbols we make and remake define us as human. Our bodies, which we interpret as meaning-makers and cultural markers, are situated at the center of who we are and how we define the current moment on earth in which we live. The anthropologists in this book set a high mark for how the future of knowing, collaborating, and interpreting the world – through culture, power, gender, and corporeal meaning – can be for the next decade. Indeed, as the world becomes smaller and more complex at the same time, our understandings of fat in a world of plenty compounded by egregious inequity and poverty will continue to demand attention. Such work that is making meaning out of experience could not be more relevant or more urgent.

Emily Mendenhall
Georgetown University

CHAPTER ONE

Introduction

"The individual is responsible for their weight. Once some-one is a high school student and they suddenly become fat, I would think 'there must be a reason' like maybe their parents or their living environment or even school is full of stress, that could be a reason. If the person is just lazy and only eating what they want, then maybe it is the parent's fault." (*Sachiko, thirty-eight-year-old mother of four in Osaka, Japan*)

"Once you gain weight, you've really seriously gotta try to work out and eat right or else you'll never lose it ... I mean, all I'd have to do is just work out and eat right. Just, you know, it's called discipline ... Yeah, I know what to do. I just don't do it right." (*Caroline, fifty-year-old woman in north Georgia, USA*)

"It depends on each person's will and perseverance. My parents or my friends can tell me, 'Look, you have to lose weight: lose weight.' But if I don't take it seriously, I'll just continue at the same weight. It depends on each person, each person's own will." (*Rosa, sixty-year-old woman in Encarnación, Paraguay*)

"I'm eating porridge in the morning. And then in the after-noon, I'll have a sandwich or – but we hardly eat taro now. Yeah, because everything is convenient. We just go to the shop and

buy the rice. And it's only two of us at home. It's so hard for
us to cook. It's laziness." (*Tofi, fifty-eight-year-old woman in
Apia, Samoa*)

Anthropologists and other scholars have long noted that biomedical
notions of health are deeply individualistic, which means individuals
are held responsible for their sickness and lauded for their health.[1]
This seems to be especially true for body size where, at least in Western contexts, an individual's achievement of certain standards of
body shape, size, and fitness are held up as personal successes. Eating disorders, for example, show us how this focus on the body as
personal achievement can have harmful consequences. The disorders
uneasily sit between behaviors widely considered positive – self-control, disciplined eating – and those that are dangerous to health, such
as self-starvation. Susan Bordo wrote in 1993 that eating disorders in
the United States were a function of young women being encouraged
to live in a culture of consumption and a culture of individual responsibility.[2] Eating disorders, she said, resulted from everyday efforts to
manage those contradictory pulls.

But what does the study of eating disorders in the United States
have to do with wider human experiences of fatness, the topic of our
book? People around the globe face everyday challenges of straddling
between "scarcity and excess" in ways that mirror those same contradictory influences that Bordo pointed out nearly thirty years ago.[3]
Global rates of obesity and related disorders like diabetes result from
contexts of scarcity of nutritious foods, while people's everyday lives
are increasingly inundated with "convenience" foods. The latter are
often also energy-dense, highly processed, and pleasure-laden foods.
Around the planet, our shared material world – the food we eat, the
bodies we live in, the environments we move through – is one that
increasingly requires many of us to make complex choices in order
to avoid harmful and dangerous foods. It's not only sugar, salt, and
fat that make our foods harmful, but the pesticides, hormones, and
pollutants that make consuming seemingly fresh fruits and vegetables
also potentially dangerous.[4] Despite the massive social, ecological,
technological, and economic changes that are so rapidly and profoundly changing our everyday lives – including where and how
we work and where and how food arrives in front of us, ready to be

eaten – many individuals around the globe operate in an environment where individual *choice* is defined as the underpinning of all global weight gain.[5] This is the focus of our ethnography: how this notion of individual responsibility, in a world of contradictory messages and pressures, explains why people around the globe of all body sizes are similarly distressed by even the possibility of gained weight.

It's impossible to understand this, however, without first considering that notions of individual responsibility are deeply rooted Western Europe and United States cultural ideas. These now permeate many institutions and practices that have come to shape how the world understands health – namely, biomedical, public health, and community development and governance efforts, as well as fitness and beauty industries.[6] Despite these shared institutional roots, anthropologists have shown how people around the world practice medicine or fitness, for example, in extraordinarily different ways.[7] This recognition of both shared historical trends and cultural differences makes cultural anthropology unique. As anthropologists, we trace global trends, including in this case the increase in weight that people experience across diverse geographies and cultures and the related increase in shared ideas about personal responsibility. We also pay attention to how personal responsibility is interpreted and explained in distinct ways around the globe. As the quotes that open this chapter show, people in many different locales associate fat with notions of lack of discipline or laziness, and find the explanation of individual responsibility persuasive. Yet, as we will also show in this book, the ways they interpret ideas around discipline, laziness, and responsibility are shaped by cultural, social, and economic context. Laziness, just like fat, doesn't mean the same thing everywhere.

Why do these cultural details of how people understand and react to "fat," extracted through the methods of cultural anthropology, matter? The persistent idea that individuals are responsible for their body size, and ultimately in control of their body size, has implications for our health. There is a growing literature that documents how feelings of being overweight, regardless of actual body size, are highly predictive for risk of depression.[8] Feeling fat-stigmatized – morally devalued by others because of failing to meet expected body norms about size – can make it harder to lose weight while increasing feelings that one should lose weight.[9] Stress, worry, and doubt about one's self-discipline may actually impact our appetites in ways that impact health. Such feelings may also cause us to avoid exercise, especially in public. Stress can trigger hormone cascades in the body that tell the body to hold onto fat and these cascades are also implicated in many chronic diseases that are thought to be associated with increased weight, such as hypertension. All these complex biocultural processes are compounded by racialized, gendered, and economic inequalities that make it more likely for marginalized communities everywhere and for people of color in countries like the United States to experience the harms associated with higher body weights and weight gain.

Related to this, pervasive ideas about individual responsibility also matter because fat stigma plays out at community and society levels as systematic discrimination of individuals (and even families and entire communities) perceived to be fat. Thus, in many places, people with extremely large bodies are systematically disadvantaged in multiple ways. In the United States, for example, we know that access to education, such as going to college, is lower for those who are pigeonholed as fat.[10] Salaries are also lower for people with very large bodies compared to the rest of the workforce.[11] The stigma of fat can build and contribute to lower economic power, including poverty. On the other hand, poverty in a country like the United States increases a person's risk of becoming fat – and of becoming fat earlier in life. There are also health implications. Fat individuals may avoid clinical care because of negative experiences with stigmatizing health-care professionals, and, as a result may, for example, receive fewer cancer screenings or influenza vaccines.[12] Fat stigma – and the closely related stigma of being perceived as more unhealthy – is also racialized in a country like the United States, where Black and brown bodies are often portrayed as naturally unhealthy and larger.[13]

The studies mentioned thus far largely focus on the contexts of Western Europe and the United States, but the ideas just described are diffusing around the world quite rapidly. An earlier preliminary study by members of our team that ultimately launched the much more detailed ethnographic investigation described in this book showed that, even in places once associated with fat positivity, people globally reported high levels of fat-stigmatizing ideas and experiences.[14] That is, by the early 2000s, it was clear to us that not only were food systems changing with accelerating globalization, but ideas about fatness were as well.

As with all processes of globalization, in the movement of ideas or foods across borders their meanings change depending on context. In American Samoa, for example, one of the sites included in that original survey study, the team members observed a curious mix of fat positive and fat negative responses, reflecting unique historical circumstances where fat could be associated with power and prestige and laziness and corruptness. In independent Samoa, where Jessica has since done detailed ethnographic data collection, she has described a mix of disparaging ideas about fatness while also observing that calling someone fat is not ordinarily an insult. Around the world we can observe a similar kind of multilayered meaning of fat.

Other ethnographic studies have shown similar heterogeneity, and in many different places. In Guatemala, for example, while people in the Highlands talked about being fat, it wasn't tied to self-identity, nor did these references include moral valences. Instead, these were self-assessments that articulated change in people's lives, mostly measured by not being able to fit into one's clothes.[15] In the largely white suburbs of Australia, while people were affected by and highly aware of the harmful stereotypes associated with fat. They also embraced a host of counter-ideas about fat that associated it with generosity or highlighted the idea of "good fats," as, for example, those associated with eating avocado. As Warin and Zivkovic put it, these communities "rationalized [fat] as a form of self-preservation and survival, strengthening, protecting and cushioning participants' bodies and figuratively, from the hard knocks of exhaustion of life."[16]

Yet, even as people maintain multiple meanings of "fatness," weight-related stigma does create vulnerabilities, vulnerabilities that can transcend generations. Maternal stress and hormonal correlates of poverty and chronic disease both impact fetuses in utero, increasing the chance of a pre-term and/or low birth weight baby, and these in turn result in the increased likelihood that the baby will struggle with weight maintenance and chronic disease risk later in life.[17] Emerging scientific evidence suggests that epigenetics – the complex early life interactions between environmental conditions and gene expression, in which certain conditions and exposures cause some genes to manifest as traits, while other genes, essentially get "turned off" – are increasingly recognized as likely relevant to explaining weight status later in life. The conditions that appear to have especially sensitive interactions with epigenetic adjustments include in utero toxic environmental exposures (including through ingested food and water), maternal dietary quality, maternal emotional trauma, and poverty and other forms of material need.[18]

Nevertheless, despite growing scientific evidence suggesting the complex, multilayered nature of weight, health professionals and the public continue to focus on individual responsibility as the driver of weight gain or loss.[19] Delving into the tenets of obesity science can help explain why this is. Emilia Sanabria argues that obesity science deflects attention away from questions about food-environment issues "not simply by the absence of good evidence but also because the existing parameters of good science cannot straightforwardly reveal such relations."[20] This is to say that the ways we as a society assign responsibility matter and these social perceptions affect our practice of science. Scientific data then goes on to influence social perceptions – in this case, worldwide. We will show in this book that experiences of worry, stress, or fear derived from shared ideas about individual responsibility were front and center on people's minds in four very different global locations. We expect they are too in many (if not most) others. This has global health, equity, and social justice implications.

We were able to explore both the remarkable shared discourse of personal responsibility and also cultural variation by using a comparative and collaborative ethnographic approach, delving into the myriad meanings and implications of "being fat" within and across different global sites. Ethnographies – cultural analyses based on doing long-term participant-observation in a specific community or context – are usually written by a single anthropologist precisely because they dig deeply into a topic based on long-term fieldwork. Our collaborative and comparative ethnography is unusual in this regard (though the older pattern is changing). Our team-based approach, still anchored in each of us having long-term familiarity with one of the sites described here, allows us to explore how the nuanced and distinct meanings of fatness for people in very different parts of the globe are increasingly *linked* by concern about weight.

When we began our collaborative fieldwork as a team of five, we did have some inkling of what we might find in our planned study of the experiences of weight across our field sites. We had all worked on these questions independently before. Our initial propositions came from talking together about what we had already been observing at each of our field sites, especially changes we had each observed in the prior decade. We all had observed changes that spoke to the widening and deepening of global concerns around the need to have a not-fat body, even as what constituted who is and who isn't fat varied across our contexts. For example, in research Alex began in Samoa in the early 1990s,[21] there was little sign of the fat worry and talk that were more common in the mainland United States at that time (where Alex was also conducting similar body image research). By the time Jessica began conducting ethnographic research in urban Samoa twenty years later, things had changed markedly.[22] Among urban women, concerns and anxieties around being fat had transformed into something about which they often spoke, even if usually in jest.

By 2015, we started talking in earnest with one another about what was happening and how we might bring the varied strands of our separate work together into a broader project that could leverage the most obvious differences between our varied field sites. Samoa had most often been described as a "fat-positive" society with historically stable food supplies, but as we just noted, that was changing quickly.[23] Japan – where Cindi has worked for decades – is a society that has long valued thin body aesthetics and careful control around food.[24] Paraguay, which Amber first visited in 2004, has intersecting concerns about undernutrition and overnutrition; these remain alongside historical memories of hunger.[25] The Southeastern United States, where Alex had first done research in the early 2000s, is frequently cited by in-country public health programs as having particular problems with obesity, healthy eating, and poverty, while also exhibiting anti-fat bias similar to that found elsewhere in the mainland United States.[26]

We also had all noticed growing anxiety around weight at other sites around the world where we had done fieldwork, even though these are not part of this study. These experiences and observations were important to our early theory building. Alex had done research with Mexican schoolchildren who were showing some of the very first indicators of a new wave of overweight in the early 1990s.[27] Sarah had conducted research in the United Arab Emirates in the 2000s, where she documented the worries articulated by young women about looking fat, precisely because there were significant social and economic repercussions for them if they did.[28] Sarah, Alex, and Amber had recently completed a four-year ethnographic study based in a bariatric (weight-loss surgery) program at a large clinic complex in the United States, where they focused on the stigma experiences and ongoing health concerns of pre- and post-operative bariatric patients.[29] Cindi had led a sociolinguistic study in the United States looking in detail at how people talk to each other about their bodies, and how that language tied to not just their physical bodies but also their social anxieties.[30]

The stories we told each other from our field sites, which we shared as we began to conceptualize this project, made it clear that even when our individual research goals were not focused on bodies, our own bodies went in and out of focus on a regular basis as we interacted with other people. In the many places we had done fieldwork, and even sometimes when we weren't studying bodies at all, people simply kept talking with us about their weight and body shape concerns in varied ways that showed how important the topic was to them. The idea that the body – what it looks like, how it acts and speaks, what it consumes, what it wears – is constantly noticed, even called out, emerged very clearly across our diverse field sites. The idea that the *fat* body is increasingly noticed and called out in specific ways is what drew us together, to explore in detail the meaning of fat bodies through our team-based ethnography.

FAT IN ANTHROPOLOGY: A BRIEF BACKGROUND

A concern for the symbolic meanings of fat bodies is nothing new to anthropology. Hortense Powdermaker drew attention to this as early as 1960, drawing a cross-cultural and historical comparison of the ways in which groups differently valued food and physical activity and how these concerns were then symbolically represented.[31] There are, in fact, many extraordinary ethnographies by solo anthropologists who did fieldwork in the 1990s that demonstrate how large bodies communicated many *positive* moral values: wealth, health, hard work, attractiveness, marriageability, social support, fertility, sexiness, and reproduction. These include Rebecca Popenoe's study of the ritualized fattening of girls in Niger to make them more marriageable; Elisa Sobo's exploration of the "sweetness" of fat in notions of womanhood in Jamaica; and Anne Becker's analysis of the ways well-fed bodies underpinned valued social relations in Fiji.[32]

More recent ethnographies have focused on the different meanings that bodies carry in places as diverse as Guatemala, Cuba, the United States, the Netherlands, Australia, India, and South Africa.[33] These more recent ethnographies have moved forward conversations around the cultural meanings of fat in important ways by highlighting histories of colonialism, political economy, and global food flows. From these varied studies we learn how social factors around race, gender, class, ethnicity, and Indigeneity shape not only who gains weight and who gets sick but also how fat is interpreted. In their focus on the ways in which the global economy shapes our bodies, works by Megan Carney, Hanna Garth, Emily Mendenhall, and Lauren Carruth showed how food insecurity and histories of food deprivation are tied to rising rates of obesity and diabetes.[34] Using the lens of structural violence, Alyshia Gálvez demonstrated the intimate links between NAFTA and rates of obesity and diabetes in Mexico.[35] Emily Mendenhall's comparative work laid out the value of taking a syndemics approach to obesity and diabetes, as she describes how, around the world, trauma influences who gets diabetes.[36] Still others, like Ashanté Reese, who explored how Black residents in Baltimore navigate and resist an unequal food distribution system, have delved into the intimate linkages between food justice and racial justice.[37]

These more recent ethnographies also grapple with tension between the meanings people apply to weight outside of a clinic or medical program and its medicalized treatment.[38] These studies suggest that national and community-based public health programs aimed at reducing obesity rates,[39] especially when taken together with a multinational diet industry and international media (and social media) messaging around the value of thinness, are likely enforcing an increasingly internalized message that weight is dangerous and must be controlled.[40] Ironically, this is happening despite the fact that the evidence linking obesity and chronic disease is highly contested. Studying the global contexts of fat also matters because we increasingly hear that obesity and fat represent a "global health crisis" that can only be avoided if people lose weight worldwide.[41] This is sometimes discussed in terms of the perception that fat people are bankrupting health-care systems with their associated expensive-to-treat diseases like diabetes.[42] For a recent example, consider the discourse in the United States during the COVID-19 pandemic around the "dangers" of obesity combined with exposure to COVID-19. This public health and medical discourse around obesity is everywhere, however, and much of it focuses on the demand that individuals change their diet and physical activity, often in the absence of clear structural and policy changes.[43] Informed by this important set of work, we began our study with the proposition that this drumbeat of messaging with a corollary lack of structural change might be one powerful way that moralizing and damaging anti-fat ideas ("fat stigma") might be spreading around the world, and even gaining traction in societies where fat bodies can be socially advantageous.[44]

TALKING ABOUT FAT

Another observation drawn from the wider body of recent ethnographic work on weight is that we need to be very thoughtful about how we talk about fat. Two common – and problematic – terms in English conversations are "fat" and "obesity."[45] In this book, we distinguish fat as a social category that describes a quality of the body. Fat can refer to the material description of all bodies. Some people have more, some have less. This contrasts to the colloquial ways that fat is used in English, with its power to accuse or shame individuals and communities; the term can be used to tease, bully, insult, and reject.[46] Many people in the United States, for example, despise or avoid the term. This is one reason why Jessica, on the first day of her undergraduate course called Food, Fat, and Fitness, asks students to shout the word out loud, together in unison. She reminds them that fat is a material, a neutral term for describing qualities or states of food or the body; fats are elements that are studied in laboratory environments.[47] Still, it's uncomfortable for most of the students. They often have to repeat the exercise for the first few weeks before everyone is able to say it without any apparent discomfort.[48]

Of course, the use of the word *fat* itself need not be invariably negative and damaging, even in potentially fat-stigmatizing contexts like US college campuses. Its power shifts depending on who uses it, for what purpose, and when and where and with whom it is used. This aligns with the way fat has often been understood by Fat

Studies scholars, who strategically use the word fat precisely because it is more typically a stigmatized and stigmatizing descriptor within general mainstream white American English.[49] Euphemisms such as "big" or "heavy" can also be used, but they then can also deflect and weaken what is really going on with the more culturally powerful descriptor, *fat*. These euphemisms also suggest that fat is so stigmatizing that it is unspeakable. Using descriptors such as heavy instead of fat does not necessarily reduce stigma because it doesn't address the underlying moral judgments. In Fat Studies, "obese" and "overweight" tend to be explicitly avoided because these terms medicalize and so judge and stigmatize bodies. This thinking has also percolated outward, influencing other disciplines, such as Women and Gender Studies.[50] The National Women's Studies Association in the United States, for example, discourages any uncritical use of Obese/Obesity in its annual conference presentations and some university presses have similar policies now in place. Fat activists and body positive activists have also made headway in very recent years in reclaiming previously derogative language, flipping the term to advocate for the notion of fat as beautiful and powerful – or at least on par with other body sizes.[51]

In this book, we do use the term "obesity." We do so to specifically reference technical medical categories that assign health values and risk to people in their roles as patients or otherwise within medical and public health systems. Medically, weight identified as "high" and adiposity identified as "excess" are measured and diagnosed using clinical classifications of Overweight and Obese. Such labels are typically made via measurements like the body mass index (BMI), a height and weight metric. BMI, the most influential metric in use globally, was designed to compare populations, not individuals, and yet it is widely used in clinical assessments.[52] In fact, the standard cut-off is arbitrary as it does not map neatly onto relative mortality risk.[53] As scholars working at the intersection of anthropology, public health, and medicine, we do find that the term is still useful in providing rough gradient understandings of population weight and indexes when we are referring to medically assigned labels related to body weight. Like other scholars situated between fields, intentional use of these terms allows us to cite and work with medical and public health practitioners worldwide who do rely on these terms.[54]

Finding shared language – with critical social scientists and health-oriented practitioners and scientists – is important because of the real-world impact that these terms have on clinical care. For example, many people in the United States who are told by others that they are fat or who themselves feel they are fat may not register as Overweight medically, based on body measurements like the BMI.[55] Moreover, those individuals who are declared in medical terms to be Obese may, in fact, be very healthy (e.g., have great metabolic health or very high muscle mass). Moreover, millions try to lose weight or to get healthy via food restrictions because of the meanings they apply to their body size and shape and not because a health-care provider told them they needed to do so for their health.[56] That said, research shows that sometimes health-care providers rely on cultural interpretations of weight and shape in their diagnoses to distinguish between weight that should be removed from the body and that which can acceptably remain. This is often a normative decision-making process, not one based on clinical cutoffs. In such a complex situation of layered meaning, shared language is important. In this book, we accordingly use "fat" most often, but we also use obese/Obese and overweight/Overweight. We use uppercase Obesity and Overweight to denote medicalized contexts.

The language of weight shapes our bodies and our worlds, and the reverse is also true.[57] In practice, there is no ideal solution for terminology because of the ways that these terms carry with them so much meaning well beyond their clinical or political application. Our book cover indexes this complexity by being as clear as we can around terms used for fat in our field sites, each with their own set of associated meanings. For example, Alex and Sarah's previous research in the United States on how young people understand weight-related terminology found the same strongly negative emotional reactions to being labeled obese as being labeled fat, if the terms were deployed to blame, shame, or negatively describe a body.[58] In other words, it was the intent behind them that bothered the young people. To be so-labeled suggests that a person not only fails to meet social norms but is also unhealthy, at risk, or even diseased. In Japan, the term for obesity is *himan*, but people do not use this word as frequently as they use *metabo* (short for *metabolic syndrome*) or a form of the word *futoru*, a verb which is best glossed as "to [become] fat." Consequently, in the parts of this text that focus on Japan, *metabo* and *futoru* appear in some instances. In Paraguay, people generally used *gordo* or *gorda*, which bluntly means "fat," to refer to themselves and others. People often said *engordarse* (to become fat) to refer to the process of gaining weight. These are the terms that appear most often in the parts of the text that focus on Paraguay. Much less often, people used the more polite medicalized term *tener sobrepeso* (to be overweight) to describe other adults, although *sobrepeso* was somewhat more commonly used to discuss children's body weights.

WHY FAT IN FOUR CULTURES (AND NOT JUST ONE)?

Working comparatively as ethnographers, our approach allows us to see what is shared in our experiences of fat in different locations in our increasingly interconnected world. It also helps reveal what is distinct to particular cultural contexts. As we said earlier, people in an increasing array of different settings are inundated with similar streams of information on the importance and apparent simplicity of weight control, healthful eating, and physical activity. "Eat less, do more!" "You can do it!" and other variations on these core messages can be found everywhere. Nevertheless, as we will explain in this book, the angst that people in very different cultural settings express around weight is not rooted in precise categories of "this is what thin looks and measures like" versus "this is what fat looks and measures like." Rather, it is embedded in the ways people classify their own and others' bodies, using categories that are surprisingly ad hoc, changeable, and slippery. Norms of what is a good and acceptable body may appear self-evident to the person (or group) relying on them, but they are, in fact, highly socially constructed and arbitrary. They also vary drastically between our field sites.

Our study also focuses on the ways ideas about fat and obesity are currently in flux when viewed globally, which mirrors what's happening with actual bodies. We know that average bodies are getting bigger at a planetary scale, with the fastest rates of increase now in lower-income countries (bodies are already big and likely to remain so in higher-income countries). This has largely been explained by scientists as due to a globalizing "nutrition transition," a worldwide shift toward a diet high in fats, sugars, and refined foods with corollary decreases in physical activity; the concept of an "epidemiological transition" refers to a related shift from a pattern characterized by a high frequency of acute infectious disease to one of chronic non-communicable diseases.[59] The novel COVID-19 pandemic certainly complicated the epidemiological profiles of many countries beginning in 2020, given it is acutely infectious and has killed and sickened billions of people around the world. The surge of cases of this one infectious disease at a particular point in time notwithstanding, it is still possible to see that the burden of chronic diseases like type 2 diabetes continue to cause more illness in a country like the United States than, for example, cholera or dysentery do. Together, these shifts add up to increases in obesity, chronic disease, and life expectancy in most parts of the world.

Such transition frameworks have been useful to researchers as we try to figure out what has happened to humans in various places around the world, what is happening, and what may happen in the future at a large scale. Transition frameworks help to compare populations, creating a sense of neutrality and comparability across many forms of difference. That sense can be misleading, just as the BMI measurements can be misleading. These frameworks have limitations when examining, as anthropologists do, particular cultural, political, and economic contexts. Transition frameworks have been critiqued for presenting an overly simplistic narrative about the global march toward modernization, problematically asserting that marginalized and minoritized communities are "not fitting" into modernity, and glossing over the effects that power (or lack thereof) has on individual and group experiences.[60] They also fail to take into account the complex interplay of infectious and chronic disease – of which the COVID-19 pandemic is one recent, glaring example.[61] In other words, they are not neutral and, sometimes, they facilitate problematic comparisons.

Based on our previous ethnographic work, we designed this study so we could theorize our way through the common patterns that linked all four sites, while capturing what makes experiences of fatness distinct in these places. This delicate balance creates an opportunity to understand how and why Western European and US ideas about personal responsibility seemingly circulate the way they do around the globe. Our own individual ethnographic studies of weight were done previously at different times, using different sets of questions, and with different agendas and methods. As we were building the framework for this shared project, we decided that what the anthropology of fat most needed was a comparative cross-cultural ethnography and we set out to develop one. This included all of us using the same shared interview protocol at all our field sites (see appendix C).

Systematic comparison allows us to see what similarities emerge between Japan, Paraguay, the United States, and Samoa, while ethnography highlights cultural variation across them, creating opportunities to speak to a continuum of obesity and fatness scholars. Our two-scale study builds on macro-level analysis (about obesity rates and fat stigma) to gather micro-level data (about everyday experiences with fatness) to make meso-level claims about what connects seemingly disparate people and places around the world. We aim to draw attention to the remarkable ways that changes in global weights are accompanied by other global phenomenon; ultimately, we aim to speak to practitioners and scholars, health professionals, and critical activists.

KEY DOMAINS

Our analytic approach to comparing across four very different field sites was focused on four theoretical domains that are part of core scholarly discussions. These were chosen because of their theoretical relevance and also because we knew from prior fieldwork that they mattered to people in all the field sites.

Domain 1: Food and Eating

The topic of food and eating is often one of the easiest areas about which to get a person talking, especially before launching into potentially sensitive conversations about bodies and weight. Food is central to the lives of all humans. It is a relatively safe topic in most places, and people also want to talk about it; food and eating often evoke positive and nostalgic memories cross-culturally. These memories connect us to those we love. Food and eating make us who we are, literally and symbolically, and in ways that are also usually acceptable to talk about in even the most casual conversations with strangers.

Our second motivation for focusing on food was that we knew from our prior work in our four research sites that people related eating to fat bodies. Every human on the planet eats and every human on the planet accumulates body fat through foods that they eat. The amounts and types of food we eat vary drastically and are inscribed with all sorts of meanings and judgments. Moreover, the scientific consensus in biomedical obesity research suggests that both the major population trends in weight gain of recent decades and the trajectories of success in individual weight loss are shaped by changes in what people eat.[62]

Consequently, research in the food domain was drawn from our own recognition that food and fat are interconnected biologically, socially, symbolically, economically, and historically. This was also informed by the work of others that came before. In Jamaica, Elisa Sobo's ethnographic work detailed how sharing food and money is essential to family life, where being thin or "stingy" were fundamentally antisocial behaviors.[63] More recently, Elizabeth Roberts reflected on the ways that food is love, and this love was created through the sharing of delightful things like *socai* in Guatemala.[64] In India, Harris Solomon delved into the complicated ways in which city dwellers in Mumbai saw interactive acts ranging from their snacks at home and trips to take-out stalls on work breaks to their exposure to urban pollutants as contributing to ill health.[65]

In our research for this book, we asked participants to describe the ways that they felt when eating and how meals had changed over time in their region, including across the generations of their own families.[66] We knew all of the communities in which we worked had experienced profound change in food patterns and availabilities in the decades after the world wars and related periods of decolonization,[67] and we outline these in each chapter. We wanted to explore these changes in detail. We also asked people about their own typical daily eating and "food labor" (growing, cooking, shopping, meal planning, food preparation). We sought to understand how these different cultural relationships with food might map onto and shape what people imagined an appropriate body size to be, as well as the appropriate ways to create or maintain it; we paid special attention to how these ideas intersected with locally relevant categories of social difference.

Domain 2: Body Ideals and Body Capital

An array of important anthropological work has made clear that bodies are socially constructed in that people build and shape their bodies to meet what they understand the cultural norms and values to be. In the United States and northwestern Europe, a range of studies have shown that people tend to draw a linear cause and effect connection between the "work" one is supposed to do that then creates a specific type of bodily product.[68] A failure to do disciplined work on the body is understood, within this framework, to produce fatness and ill health, and to be the result of an individual being lazy or neglectful.[69]

Anne Becker's work in the Pacific nation of Fiji in the 1980s showed that people saw bodies as reflections of the failings of the family or the community, not of the individual. Her work was pivotal in forcing scholars to think about cultural norms and deeply engrained assumptions that saw the individual as the unit of analysis and conflated particular types of productivity with morality. Her work also revealed very different ideas about what constituted a "good body" in Fiji. Thinness meant lack of care or concern, and the failure of the family to "feed up" its members and take care of them. Becker's more recent work has documented how these values have changed, as younger Fijians now must combine intergenerational ideas about the need for full bodies with newer (media carried) ideas about the importance of body control and body work.[70] We have ourselves also seen signs of the same trends underway in Samoa and beginning in Paraguay.[71] By contrast, Japan has long been cited as a location where women in particular have been expected to control food and body to sometimes extreme levels in order to adhere to appropriate feminine norms. A similar situation has prevailed in the American South for some time as well.[72] Thus, we included a set of questions that examined how people perceived their bodies in relation to local social expectations, including the benefits and costs of working to meet the expectations.

We also knew from others' ethnographic work in the anthropology of fat that the body can be a very powerful social accelerator – or impediment – for advancement.[73] For example, Alexander Edmond's ethnography of young women living in *favelas* (informal settlements) and aspiring to move up the socioeconomic ladder in Brazil showed how their chances to marry well and/or get a better job were embedded in their capacity to look attractive, including in ways that increasingly echoed the US media's ideal (at the time) that emphasized tiny waists and big breasts.[74] As a key ethnographic contrast, Rebecca Popenoe's ethnography of nomadic communities in Niger documented the ways in which large bodies, rolling with carefully cultivated fat, helped young women secure desirable marriages in a very specific community, place, and time.[75] Thus, our research aimed to unravel how local opportunities, economics, and concerns around "making a good life" shaped people's relationships to their own and others' fat across the different contexts.

Additionally, we were interested in identifying gendered differences in body ideals, paying particular heed to the ways that age, motherhood, and sexuality all might influence body ideals and become embodied in women.[76] By embodied, we mean the ways that cultural values and processes become inscribed as physical traits on the body.[77] Through the elicitation of nuanced body ideals, including asking people about specific body parts, we aimed to draw out the different ways that shape, texture, and composition were incorporated into considerations about fat. This produced examples of how not all fat is bad, but rather that fat that is out of place and uncontrolled is often the perceived problem.[78] Our work was also informed by feminist literature that explicates how fat or thin bodies might be linked to certain gender, labor, class, or age categories.[79] We focused both on the ways that people expected that bodies would be interpreted by others and how they experienced their own bodies.

Domain 3: Disease and Physical Health in Large Bodies

Much of the current scientific discussions of obesity emphasize that it is a medical issue, focusing on its association with "expensive-to-treat" chronic diseases like diabetes and cardiovascular disease. This focus is likely what a patient will hear from a health professional when they become classified in clinical terms as Overweight or Obese. This is also the focus of most public health programs that collect data and development interventions aimed at reducing weight and chronic disease. In this way, Obesity has become a medical condition (one where the "O" gets capitalized), which has rewritten the everyday experiences and reality of many people identified as Obese. Although there is also clear medical evidence that not all fat people are diseased and that many thin people can have poor metabolic health, these findings have been less popular and fewer people – whether they work in health care or not – are familiar with them.

In recent decades, as public alarm over obesity has risen in almost all countries, some scholars have pointed to the social construction of the obesity epidemic as a form of moral panic.[80] Biocultural anthropologist Tina Moffat argues a social constructionist point of view is valuable in demonstrating the limitations of medicalizing obesity, which include "the individualization of the phenomenon resulting in victim blaming; the conflation of the categories Overweight and Obese; the promotion of the epidemic for capitalist exploitation; and the stigmatization of women, ethnic minorities, and those of low socioeconomic status (SES)."[81] These critiques help us understand how medical framing may enhance the emotional suffering of individuals and detract from the structural and environmental factors that shape who gets sick and who is shielded from sickness. Moffat argues that both parties – critical scholars and medical professionals – "must begin to hear each other's views."[82]

In writing this book, we aimed to walk this middle path by exploring the processes by which people themselves may connect fat and health. We aim to explore how people explain fat or thin bodies: who and what do they see as being responsible for body size and shape? This question is based on the idea that people's rights and access to resources and social networks are defined and curtailed by their biological status, including being perceived or classified as obese or diseased.[83] We also ask, how do people understand the environmental causes of weight changes and chronic sickness in their community? This question is based on the idea that people in their own communities are experts on the causes of local sicknesses and ultimately the solutions to them.[84] To explore this idea, we asked people to explain how they thought about large bodies in relation to diverse genders, ages, and financial backgrounds.

Domain 4: Stigma and Fat Talk

In Alex and Amber's prior pilot survey research in American Samoa, the United States, and Paraguay, they demonstrated that fat stigma – the social devaluing of people with large bodies – was evident in all three sites. While negative judgments appeared in all three locations, Paraguayans showed a unique (in that study) pattern of *saying* "fat is bad," but *thinking* "fat is no big deal."[85] Japan, as we have already noted, also has a clear history of fat stigma. As a result, we suspected that negative reactions to fat, ranging from sideways glances to outright teasing, could possibly be happening in all of our field sites.

Such exhibition of fat stigma is potentially a very sensitive topic to investigate for a variety of reasons. It involves exploring people's often unpleasant social experiences with fat and their own sense of how well they fit (or don't fit) with prevailing body norms. Many people – and this applies in many cultural contexts, although certainly it is not universal – find this deeply and even threateningly personal. Asking about anti-fat beliefs or actions is also potentially sensitive, however, because it involves asking people about the ways they negatively judge others. The hope in such moments is that – if the ethnographer has done a good job building trust and rapport – people will be more willing to discuss such tricky topics. We didn't necessarily assume complete accuracy, however. Following the anthropological truism that what people say they do might not coincide with what they actually do,[86] we asked people to share specific instances of feeling pride, shame, and ambivalence about bodies, based on the fact that specific examples would increase people's recall.

Communicating judgment with comments and with body language can have different social effects, depending on where you are and with whom you are speaking. For example, in the United States, judgmental body comments might be shrugged off in some contexts (like on an all-male basketball court), but could strongly shape body anxieties in other contexts (like on a mixed-use beach). The effects of a comment about size will also be felt differently in Paraguay versus Japan. This is why conducting participant-observation within our research sites was so important. It helps us understand what forms of fat judgment people noticed, reacted to, and condoned. It shows how different contexts allow for alternative ways of reacting to, coping with, and negotiating these judgments.

We knew from Amber's prior work in Paraguay, for example, that people publicly teased individuals with large bodies harshly, and we knew from Jessica's prior work in Samoa that laughing about the bodies of others was a basic widespread form of humor within many social interactions. People use language to negotiate and mediate all aspects of their lives – food use, body ideals and norms, and body sizes are no exception. This meant that we needed to pay careful attention to language. We accordingly also considered the fine details of how people talked to others about their bodies and fat, with whom, and where these conversations occurred. We collected fat jokes and paid close attention to who thought they were funny, who pretended to think they were funny, and who did not find them funny at all and said so.

ORGANIZATION OF THIS BOOK

The chapters that follow provide details of what we did in each of our four field sites, how we used our interview protocols, and what we found across the four theoretical domains just described. In chapter 2, we explore our protocols and methods, paying particular attention to the collaborative and comparative aspects of our ethnographic research (although the fully detailed exploration of our methods is located in the appendices). You will also find background information for each of the sites in chapter 2. In chapters 3 to 6, we each take turns discussing our field sites. As we remarked at the beginning of this introduction, our book is an exploration of how disparate people in very different locations around the world tackle the question of what it means to be fat in today's world, how one becomes fat, and what sorts of consequences subsequently emerge. Cindi focuses on the implications of these questions in Osaka, Japan, in chapter 3; Alex and Sarah do the same in the context of north Georgia in the United States in chapter 4; Amber does so in Encarnación, Paraguay, in chapter 5; and Jessica explores these in the context of Apia, Samoa, in chapter 6. In chapters 7 and 8, we again pull our lens back to discuss the big picture, tracing similarities across our field sites and the implications of these. Our appendices and notes are designed to be of use to those who want more information on our methods.

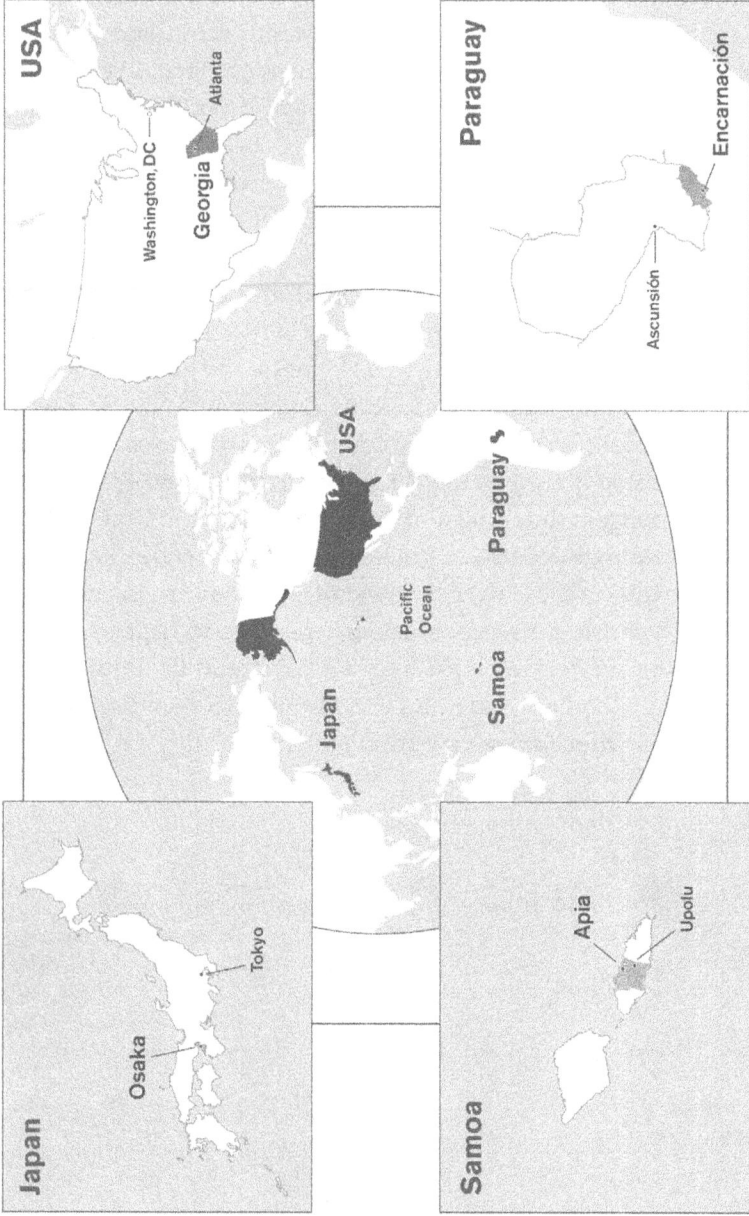

Figure 2.1. A map of the field sites

CHAPTER TWO

How and Where We Did the Study

This study employs an explicitly cross-cultural comparative ethnographic perspective. For any reader unfamiliar with anthropology, a little more explanation might be useful. Anthropology, a discipline interested in the study of humanity, has long appreciated the advantages of global, comparative studies of human beliefs, behaviors, and social organization. The detailed process of "doing" ethnography – of immersing oneself in a community, culture, and place and attempting to systematically describe what people do, believe, and say within that context – requires prolonged, careful study at the micro level. Much anthropological knowledge is therefore built slowly over time by comparing and contrasting across distinct studies of different places, incrementally building broader theory via the case-by-case accumulation of data. Doing cultural comparison as part of an explicit and carefully planned research design, by directly comparing cases to examine how they vary and overlap, can be time intensive and laborious, and most ethnographers delve into just one or two sites in their career. To overcome these difficulties, we used a collaborative approach to comparative ethnography in this study.

A COMPARATIVE ETHNOGRAPHIC APPROACH

Ethnography is the defining method of cultural anthropology. It requires long-term engagement and is rooted in participant-observation, a method that involves learning to live with and as the people in the research study do. It is also based on localized understandings, the establishment of relationships of trust with local research participants, and learning the language(s) and lexicon(s) of the community studied. Ethnography is often inductive (theorizing "from the ground up") but can also be deductive (theorizing based on existing research and scholarly literature). It requires embeddedness in communities. Ethnography thus rests on a set of methods practiced by the anthropologist-ethnographer while following the expertise of research participants and partners.[1]

Cross-cultural ethnography is singularly powerful in parsing out what shared experiences, norms, and behaviors are like in different communities. One of the most famous examples of a cross-cultural ethnographic study is Brigitte Jordan's 1992 book, *Birth in Four Cultures*.[2] Jordan's widely read study expanded the idea of using ethnography as the point of anthropological comparison. Jordan did her fieldwork at four disparate sites: the Yucatan, Holland, Sweden, and the United States. She observed births as they took place in each of these settings, describing the ways that the mother and the people attending her understood the biological and social processes involved in childbirth. Births across the four sites ultimately all produced babies but the explanations for the particular birthing behaviors (sitting vs. lying down during labor, foods that are consumed or eschewed, the role of the father in the birth, etc.) and decisions differed vastly across the sites. The book was valuable in demonstrating that all human processes, no matter how biologically universal, are fundamentally informed and transformed by social processes.

Direct comparison of cases ethnographically allows us to look at complex, large-scale phenomena. Consider the 1963 *Six Cultures Study*.[3] Through a collection of directly comparable observational data from the United States (Massachusetts), the Philippines (Ilocos), Japan (Okinawa), Kenya (Gusii), Mexico (Juxtlahuaca), and India (Khalapur), this study contrasted and compared how parents across these six distinct societies reared children to be fully functioning adults according to the norms and rules of their communities. In doing so, it seeded an important new understanding: the way children are raised shapes their adult personalities. While the authors' interpretation of the findings continues to be debated, the clarification (and the empirical evidence supporting the clarification) that culture could directly shape how whole groups of adults interacted with the world around them was an important one at the time.

Another exciting trend has been a renaissance in cross-cultural methods, including comparative ethnography.[4] The book that arguably kicked off this renaissance was the 2009 comparative ethnography *The Secret: Love, Marriage, and HIV*, in which the authors explored marital and extramarital sex in five sites in Nigeria, Uganda, Mexico, Vietnam, and Papua New Guinea.[5] Another important example was a study, led by anthropologist Svea Closser, which examined vaccine refusal as part of the Global Polio Eradication Initiative.[6] Similarly, Emily Mendenhall's 2019 book, *Rethinking Diabetes: Entanglements with Trauma, Poverty, and HIV,* draws on her ethnographic work in Chicago (US), Delhi (India), Soweto (South Africa), and Nairobi (Kenya) to explore how diabetes is a synergistic epidemic that co-occurs with poverty, HIV, depression, trauma, and other health conditions.[7] As these examples show, the space where anthropology meets global health is particularly fertile ground for cross-cultural comparative ethnographies. Cross-cultural work is further supported by recent methodological advances, such as those put forward in the 2020 volume *Comparing Cultures: Innovations in Comparative Ethnography*.[8]

WHY THESE FOUR SITES?

An important element of cross-cultural research design is choosing sites that help us explore similarities and differences in how people think about everyday aspects of life.[9] These kinds of explorations allow us to better understand the specific social, cultural, historical, and political underpinnings to everyday assumptions, attitudes, and ways of being in the world that – without a different set of reference points – people often assume are universal, not context-specific. We chose four sites that showed different national Obesity rates and also evidence of different articulated fat stigma. By this,

Table 2.1. Non-communicable disease rates*

	Japan	USA	Paraguay	Samoa
Proportional mortality (%)				
Cardiovascular disease	27	30	29	34
Cancers	30	22	16	15
Chronic respiratory diseases	9	9	3	5
Diabetes	1	3	7	9
Injuries	5	7	12	7
Other NCDs	15	24	20	18
Population level rates (%)				
Diabetes	10	9	7	23
Raised blood pressure	27	16	22	22

*For a list by country, see https://www.who.int/nmh/countries/en/#U.

Table 2.2. Rationale for site selection

	Lower obesity	Higher obesity
Less fat-stigmatizing	Encarnación, Paraguay	Apia, Samoa
More fat-stigmatizing	Osaka, Japan	North Georgia, USA

we mean that we selected these four sites because they differed from one another in terms of the average size of the bodies and disease profiles of people living there (see table 2.1) and also in terms of judgmental cultural attitudes toward fat bodies compared to thinner ones (see table 2.2).

Throughout this book, we present the information for each site based on a continuum of the stigmatization of fat while also noting whether the site also exhibits high/low Obesity rates based on the World Health Organization's (WHO) categories. In this framework, Japan is the most stigmatizing, followed by the United States, then Paraguay, and then Samoa. A continuum model is useful because it acknowledges that while fat stigma may be high in some places, in day-to-day life, it may not be universally experienced. In other words, though there are dominant discourses that enforce fat stigma, individual experience shaped by localized cultural and social norms may resist those dominant discourses, or at least express some ambivalence about their dominance.[10]

A FIELD SITE OVERVIEW

Japan

Japan is a highly industrialized nation, with most of its people living in large cities. It boasts one of the lowest adult Obesity rates in the world, at just 4.3 per cent, and the rate of Overweight is 27.2 per cent. In part, these low rates reflect the ongoing influence of the traditional Japanese diet in everyday life, a diet characterized by lots of fresh vegetables and high quality proteins like fish. Japanese participants consistently expressed skepticism on learning that they were part of a study of fat/obesity, saying, "Japanese people aren't obese like people in the United States are." Indeed, since the middle of the last century, Japan has been identified as a country of extreme thin-idealism.

In what at first appears completely contradictory to the data just cited, however, the government of Japan announced in the early 2000s that the nation was in the midst of a burgeoning Obesity crisis, basing this assertion on a different interpretation of BMI measurements (more on this later in the book). The government has taken dramatic steps to do something about this identified crisis. In 2008, the Japanese parliament passed the *"metabo* law" that specified the allowable waistline of those employed in companies: 33.5 inches for men and 35.4 inches for women. Individuals who are categorized as being at risk for metabolic diseases face the prospect of special counseling and education classes, and companies with too many wide-waisted employees risk stiff fines.

Osakan society, like that of Japan generally, is defined by highly delineated gender roles and publicly inflexible notions of masculinity and femininity. Once married, urban women are expected to focus their attention on the home and family; nevertheless, the vast majority of women work at least part time. Men are expected to focus their attention on work, earning money, and supporting the family financially. These sharp social delineations permeate how people understand and react to fatness in their everyday lives. Fat (*futotteru*) for men is considered somewhat understandable, given the long sedentary hours and poor quality meals men are expected to face as earners, but people feel women's fat is harder to excuse. Women, too, are often held responsible for managing their husband's (and children's) weight. As Osakans collectively gain weight in the years ahead (an upward trend that is based on current in-country predictions), gender will matter greatly in how responsibility and blame for those national trends and personal pounds are allocated.

The United States

The United States is one of several "high Obesity" countries in the world today (using the admittedly problematic WHO and Centers for Disease Control categories assessing the epidemiology of Obesity). National Obesity rates are 36.2 per cent, while Overweight rates are 67.9 per cent. The numbers only tell a partial story, however, because the real power of the United States when it comes to topics around fat/obesity is its power as an international norm. The United States is a trope, one that is repeatedly returned to in discussions of fatness, obesity epidemics, and the political economy of health. We work in a variety of field sites, and the United States often comes up as a bar-setting case for understanding obesity. Interestingly, this encompasses both critical discussions of fat stigma and medicalized discussions of obesity. Thus, the concept of the United States as a highly fat stigmatizing country full of fat people is pervasive worldwide but also powerful in-country. Patriotic United States nationals who don't buy into "ugly American" stereotypes across other identity markers readily accept the idea that, as one participant in Georgia put it, "The US is the fattest country in the history of the world." While this is not true – the United States is not actually the fattest country in the world, nor is it the most fat-stigmatizing – other countries have perhaps not captured the global imaginary in quite the same way.

What the United States also does very well is to provide a clear example of the stark contradictions that pervade discussions of fatness, inequality, stigma, and health epidemics. Policy-makers have not systematically supported policies and infrastructure to make healthy food more accessible and to facilitate active daily lifestyles. This has made much of the US landscape "obesogenic" (obesity-producing), especially for citizens who lack financial and social capital. People in the United States have also not substantially changed their thinking that equates large bodies with lack of discipline and self-control.[11] Ironically, both stem from a set of cultural values that place responsibility for health, wellness, and good citizenship on the individual. The much-loved phrase "Pull yourself up by your bootstraps" (a feat that is technically impossible, no matter how tiny your size) is thus rewritten onto discussions of fatness.

The United States, including Georgia, has had precipitously increasing rates of adult Obesity since World War II. There are widespread efforts at the policy level (by which we mean federal and state governments, school systems, and public health programs) to encourage people in the United States to eat more healthy food and to exercise regularly. Obesity rates may be plateauing as a result – but they aren't reversing. In Georgia, as with the rest of the United States, Obesity has been increasingly associated with poverty and other forms of disadvantage. Across the United States, the lower the socio-economic status, the higher the risk of Obesity. Despite how common Obesity is (roughly one-third of adults), fat-related discrimination remains common as well.

Paraguay

Paraguay, a small landlocked country in South America's Southern Cone, is one of the most explicitly fat-stigmatizing sites documented in the world.[12] People have no qualms about telling someone else that they are too fat, need to lose a few pounds, or just generally look terrible. This frankness is unlike most other fat-stigmatizing sites around the world, where people register high rates of fat stigma but tend to downplay such views when they speak. In sites like the United States and Japan, people are more likely to *think* fat is immoral, undisciplined, and disgusting but are less likely to *say* so, especially directly to someone they identify as fat. In Paraguay, in contrast, people may joke, tease, or criticize fat out loud, but psychological tests indicate Paraguayans generally do not have anti-fat attitudes.[13] Later in the book, we'll have much to say about the ways this unusual combination plays out in day-to-day interactions in Encarnación.

Paraguay is unusual in other ways, too. It has been called the "happiest nation in the world," a country where people report feeling very positive and having a strong sense of community, despite historic and current political economic challenges.[14] One component of this positivity stems from Paraguayans' commitment to their unique cultural heritage, including speaking the indigenous Guarani language (an official national language), drinking *terere* (cold *yerba mate* tea) in communal sharing circles, preparing and eating Paraguayan foods (like *chipa*, a cheesy bread), and nurturing the sociocultural institutions that undergird these traditions. In Paraguayan *terere* drinking circles, fat shaming and offering social support go hand in hand, as teasing and helping are equally embraced as culturally valued practices.[15] While it is common for people in Paraguay to be Overweight (53.5 per cent), Obesity rates are relatively low (20.3 per cent). Paraguayans recognize this, often saying that Paraguayan bodies are normal and rarely embody extremes of thinness or fatness.

In Encarnación, Obesity is on the rise but very high body weights are rare. Though people are increasingly working in sedentary jobs, the city is highly walkable and it is common to walk to do errands, visit friends, or just to go for a stroll. As life becomes faster-paced, fewer families prepare homemade meals and fast food restaurants are ubiquitous. Gender norms are shifting, as families are increasingly likely to have dual-income earners and men have become more involved in food preparation (including shopping). Nevertheless, responsibilities for childcare and cooking do fall disproportionately to women.

Samoa

Samoa, an island nation in Oceania, has seen a rapid rise in weight over the past half century, reflecting regional trends whereby Oceanic peoples have experienced the largest increases in adult BMI per decade in the world.[16] This development was rapid: between 1980 and 2010, out of all the regions in the world, the countries in Oceania had the greatest increase in BMI. In rural Samoa, from 1978 to 1991, Obesity increased in men by 297 per cent and in women by 115 per cent.[17] Seventy per cent of all death in the region can be linked to weight-related diseases, and in similar places like Tonga, life expectancy has fallen in recent years as a result.[18] Samoa, in particular, has long been studied by scientists as a purported "natural experiment" for understanding epidemiological/nutritional transitions.[19] Some of the first studies of the current epidemiological transition came from Samoa because the population is ethnically and culturally homogeneous but geographically distributed across varying locations, as Samoans are divided between independent

Samoa and American Samoa and there are large diasporic communities in the United States, New Zealand, Australia, and Fiji.[20] Moving from Samoa to American Samoa to Hawaii to the mainland United States means an upward weight trajectory if one happens to be Samoan. As early as the 1950s, Samoans began gaining weight as the islands became more integrated into the global economy. With that integration came dietary changes, increased migration, urbanization, and changes in labor from agricultural work to military deployment or white-collar work. Obesity levels among Samoan populations are lowest among those still living in independent Samoa, but are still high: rates of Obesity are 47.3 per cent, while rates of Overweight are 77.6 per cent.[21]

Diets in Samoa once were largely derived from family agriculture, including starches like taro, breadfruit, and banana, which were supplemented with coconut and other fruits like papaya.[22] This diet included occasional meat consumption, which was often fatty but infrequent and was complemented by agricultural labor to offset to'ona'i (calorie-dense Sunday meals). In Samoa, overall calorie consumption remains steady but agricultural labor (and activity in general) has decreased, leaving those in cities especially at risk for rapid weight gain.[23] Moreover, dietary composition has changed dramatically, as diets now follow a pattern seen all over the Pacific: reliance on imported, highly processed, high-fat, high-sugar, high-salt foods. This is especially true in the urban areas. Samoa recently "graduated" (in the World Bank rankings) from a lower-income to a middle-income country. Samoan society is highly hierarchical, and food is part of how those social hierarchies are created and maintained. Historically, fatty, salty, and sugary foods were reserved for those of the highest status like *matai* (chiefs) or church leaders; these leaders also were shielded from the intensive labor needed to sustain extended families in an agricultural economy. Thus, social power and large bodies went together in Samoan society historically.

GENDER IN OUR STUDY

Gender was a foundational focus for our study because gendered social roles differ across the four sites in ways relevant to how people understand and respond to fat. Therefore, this comparative ethnography builds on the feminist tradition of placing power dynamics and gender at the center of analysis.[24] We focus here on people with dominant gender identities (women/men), rather than those with non-binary or genderqueer identities, in order to unravel the way fat is experienced in mainstream and institutionalized gender discourses. Based on our prior research experience and the existing literature, we knew from the outset of this study that historically, women have been more harshly judged on their weight than have men across all our sites (even as this is expressed in distinct and historical ways across our sites); they also face harsher criticism in their roles as parents than do their male counterparts.[25] In higher-income nations, there are higher rates of anorexia and other eating disorders among women, women spend more on weight-loss interventions, and women are judged more for body size and shape when being considered as romantic and career prospects.[26] We also knew from the outset that our own gender identities – we are a team of five white women anthropologists – would inevitably affect the course the interviews took.

The contrast between the women and men we interviewed is important here, both because women are more affected by social judgments around weight and because women interviewees were more likely to delve into gendered disparities with us, the women interviewers. Men are increasingly affected by weight stigma, but age mitigates the degree of this effect.[27] In Samoa and the United States, women are significantly more likely to be Overweight than men. In Japan, men are more likely to be Overweight than women. In Paraguay, men and women are similar. In Japan, dominant gender norms dictate that women manage the domestic sphere while men work, which creates different eating cycles and perceived responsibilities around food – and women face relatively more pressure to maintain smaller waistlines. In the United States, even in dual income (heteronormative) households, women still shoulder more responsibility for feeding and managing the family (especially if there are children in the home), and although thin idealization increasingly affects both young women and young men, women still face more scrutiny concerning their bodies. In other words, each context shapes how gender affects experiences around weight. Local contexts matter.

COLLECTING AND ANALYZING DATA IN FOUR SITES

Participants in our study were adult women and men from within the communities just described who were willing to talk with us about health, food, fitness, and their bodies. Our study uses a purposive sample in each site, in which each of us selected our interviewees based on pre-specified targets of gender and age. We sampled at least twelve women (six under forty-five years old; six over forty-five years old) in each site, a sample size that is enough to identity themes; this also enabled us to make some important comparisons. We included at least four men in each site: two spouses of women under forty-five, and two spouses of women over forty-five.

We were also inspired by theoretical sampling – a technique in grounded theory in which participants are chosen because they can help bring novel theoretical insights to the study – to recruit people with a range of experiences with fat. Some participants identified as fat; some identified as not-fat-but-needing-to-lose-weight; and some identified as fit or skinny. The overwhelming majority registered some degree of dissatisfaction with at least some aspect of their bodies, accompanied by expressed feelings of "needing to be better" (i.e., exercise more, eat more home-cooked meals, eat less packaged highly processed food).

Analytically, it is important to note that our comparisons from place to place reflect the situation within very localized sites. Although our four sites are situated in distinct nations – Japan, Paraguay, the United States, and Samoa – we specifically worked in the suburban and peri-urban areas around Osaka, Japan; the small city of Encarnación, Paraguay; the peri-urban and rural areas north of Atlanta, Georgia, in the United States; and the capital city of Apia in Samoa. We did participant-observation to better understand the food landscapes and physical activity environments in each of our sites. The fieldnotes we amassed based on this participant observation also formed part of our data.

Using well-established techniques for theme identification, we analyzed our data for metaphors, idioms, and other indicators of shared meaning. When we met together to find the places in our data that diverged and converged, we used a qualitative technique called meta-theme analysis (described in detail in appendix B). This method is designed to capture broad meanings, encompassing multiple themes inductively in qualitative data. We used metatheme analysis as a basis for systematic comparisons and synthesis across and within our datasets, and as a starting place for our ethnographic writing process.

WRITING COLLABORATIVE CROSS-CULTURAL ETHNOGRAPHY

Writing ethnography entails translating lived experiences into stories that resonate with readers, who are often from vastly different worlds than the ones depicted in the writing. While historically less common, it has now become routine for anthropologists to take seriously the call to visibly insert themselves into their writing and research. The point of doing this is to acknowledge how the researchers' positionality – that is, the collection of identities like race, gender, class, and sexuality that shape a person's sense of self and life chances – influences the kinds of questions the researchers ask, as well as the kinds of answers they receive.[28] Ethnography is a practice of dialogue, so including the anthropologist's voice is essential. This change in approach has been pivotal in acknowledging, and reforming, anthropology's historical role in colonial endeavors.[29] In this book, we lay out some features of our own positionalities that shaped our project.

How people react to us as researchers inhabiting gendered bodies is quite different across the sites and affects our relationships to our participants in many complicated ways – even though all five of us are working mothers with steady academic jobs, white women who do not consistently identify as fat, and US passport holders. In Japan, Cindi, who is tall by US standards, is perceived to be large for a woman; consequently, at meals, she is served extra-large portions with the expectation that she will easily clean her plate. In Paraguay, Amber regularly gets side-eyed and teased for hogging the salad and avoiding meats and breads at meals, because she is correctly understood to be attempting to avoid weight gain in ways that withdraw her from communal eating and sharing. In Samoa, Jessica found people eager to feed her in her initial years there. Later, when she returned at a higher weight, with a baby accompanying her to interviews, her body better satisfied her Samoan friends and contacts. When she lost some weight, they re-expressed concern. In the United States, "average" Sarah and

Alex didn't stand out at all in the mostly white enclaves of Georgia where their research was situated – until they opened their mouths and a West Coast (of the United States) variety of English (Sarah) and a New Zealand English language variety (Alex) issued forth.

In our discussions together, we paid attention to how all these types of factors shaped what we saw and learned, and what we missed or ignored. In doing so, we follow the lead of feminist anthropologists who have critiqued the disciplinary history that assumed a supposedly neutral, lone fieldworker.[30] Historically, the role of anthropologists' own presuppositions and positions (usually white, college educated, and male) in shaping what they saw and heard went unnoticed.[31] Feminist ethnographers were some of the first to show how ethnography often told a one-sided story: that of culture, economy, and politics from the perspective of men[32] as an undifferentiated group. Feminist ethnographers began to demonstrate this absence by studying the lives of small communities of women, giving particular attention to various forms of marginalization related to race, class, sexuality, and other forms of difference.[33] Another feature of feminist ethnography is acknowledging and reflecting upon power dynamics between the anthropologist and her interlocutors,[34] something that we kept in our minds as we developed our protocol. Our aim to tell the stories and analyze them in ways that challenge the social inequities revolving around who gets sick, who gains weight, and who experiences stigma is informed by feminist research approaches as well.

When it came to the actual writing of the book manuscript, we again had to think about representation and resonance, but among multiple authors. While today, most ethnographers write in the first person to make clear their own positions through the consistent use of "I saw/we felt" statements, when writing collaboratively about independently conducted fieldwork, a first-person narrative becomes unwieldy and arguably somewhat misleading. This text is therefore written in the third person consistently across all the data-driven, field site–specific chapters. We did write chapters 1, 2, 7, and 8 together as well as the appendices and these are written in the first-person plural (see figure 2.2). We also take this process of writing as an example of feminist practices of collaboration, where just as fieldwork has historically been defined by the solo model, ethnographic writing has historically privileged an individual position as well. The "I-witnessing"

With the exception of the Samoa site, all participants recognized Americans as overweight. For participants in the Japan site this also mapped more generally onto white Westerners, whereas in the Paraguay site Brazilians and Argentinians were identified as fat others. In the Georgia site, the south was understood to be not like the rest, and thus outsider, due to it frequency of obesity among the southern population. In the Samoa site, people in positions of power including pastors and government officials were understood to be large bodied and, in this way, occupied outsider status from everyday people.

Comment [24]: But this isn't really outsider status. Fat isn't an outsider status to Americans and I don't think this quite works in GA.

Taken together, the differences across the sites demonstrate that fat could be a marker of insider or outsider status—depending on social context. People's socio-economic status was also recognized, cross-culturally, as affecting their ability to adopt healthy diets and lose weight. The sites demonstrate that the idea of cultural belonging in contrast to 'foreignness' could at times be linked closely with weight but were not solely determined by weight. The body is a complex site of meaning-making. And, the meaning that a body makes or creates is complexified by the social context. As societies are always in transition, body weights and accompanying norms are in flux; consequently, the relationships among fat, class, and belongingness in each of these four sites were very fluid.

Amber Wutich 10/15/19 12:35 PM
Comment [25]: Oh God, I am making the circle hands. It's all complex, and I have no clarity in my thinking…It just circles and circles and I haven't had time to unravel it…Sob!

Microsoft Off. 10/20/19 5:54 PM
Comment [26]: See if you think I've done any better or not. Double sob.

Table 7.6b: Exemplars of Cross-Cutting Theme: Fat marks Insider/Outsider Status

Study Site	Exemplar Quotes
Osaka, Japan	"Compared to Japanese people, French people are fat. They don't care if their bellies hang out or their belly button shows; French people are fatter than Japanese

Figure 2.2. Collaborative writing – A screenshot of our collective writing process

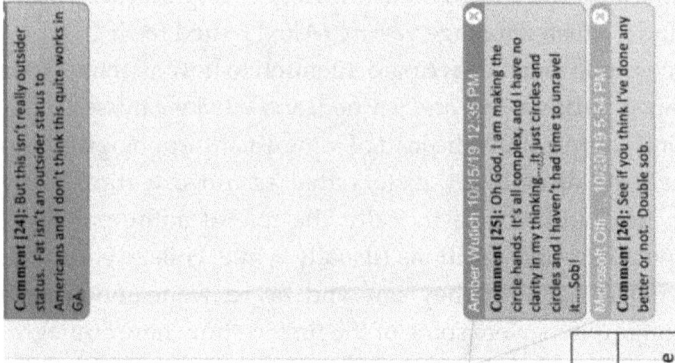

approach venerates individual intellectual efforts, while fieldwork and writing are always social processes that involve many people.[35] In our work, we write to de-emphasize individual voices and instead emphasize our shared, co-constructed forms of analyses.[36]

THE ETHICS OF STUDYING FAT

Studying fat poses some ethical challenges.[37] These pitfalls are based in pervasive and taken-for-granted stigma levied against individuals (and even whole communities) who are socially identified as fat. Most of the perspectives we hear and see in popular US and Japanese media about fat, for example, are not based on the insights or input of those who actually identify as fat. Moreover, discrimination against people on the basis of size is currently legal in many states in the United States, as it is in Japan both historically and also contemporarily via the *metabo* regulations. This means mistreatment based on size is often normalized to the point where it isn't even noticed in these places. Anyone who studies fat has a responsibility to write in ways that include a full awareness of this and limit the misuse of their research.

Moreover, it isn't just large-bodied people who are judged. Stigma often gets levied against individuals, especially women, who are deemed to be overly preoccupied with their appearance or overly sensitive about their weight across all four of our contexts. Accordingly, inviting anyone to be in a study about weight and asking them to talk about their bodies can reinforce anxieties or stigma. It can bring memories of social rejections, or hunger related to food insecurity, or uncomfortably challenge how people see themselves. Working in the context of trusting relationships and long-term commitment to our field sites, we were careful to engage participants on their terms, cognizant of their time and expertise. We explained the study thoughtfully, and focused on discussing the domains we would explore – eating, everyday life, judgment, and so on – rather than just talking about fat. We also aimed to let participants control the tone of the interviews and related conversations as they developed. We had a structured interview protocol, but even within such a framework, it was important to frame and introduce the protocol in a way that made people feel free (1) not to answer at all or (2) to curtail responses if an area felt too sensitive.

A concern with presenting people in ways with which they would be comfortable was part of the decision-making about how we represent them in this text. By focusing on weight as part of a larger lifeworld, we highlight *universally* shared worry and concern while exploring cultural differences, attempting to work against the various forms of marginalization and inequities that revolve around body size. We do this by telling stories in ways that help readers see our participants as complex people moving through a complicated world. Any social research into weight, we believe, has a moral imperative to do this.[38]

CHAPTER THREE

Futotteru (Fat) in Osaka, Japan

On a sweaty summer day in the late 1980s, Cindi went on an outing with her friend, Yōko, and Yōko's family. They were getting into the family's car for a day trip to see Shinto shrines in the old Japanese city of Kyoto. Yōko's father pointed at his daughter's legs. "*Oi! Daikon ashi ya na,*" he declared, "Hey! You have daikon legs!" Daikon, the long tapering white radish, wide at the top, but narrow at the bottom, is found in many pickled condiments and meals on Japanese tables. Even though Cindi was still learning Japanese at the time, she instantly recognized that having one's legs compared to a thick root vegetable was not a good thing. The closest American English equivalent would be telling someone that they have "cankles" (*calf* and *ankle* blended to spell *cankle*). At the time, nobody replied to Yōko's father's comment. His less-than-flattering statement hung in the air, unaddressed.

Decades later, now fluent in Japanese, Cindi was again in Osaka, this time doing the research for this book. A different friend, Reiko, made a notable confession. Several weeks before, Cindi had interviewed her about fat, health, and fitness as they play out in everyday life in Japan. In responding to the interview questions about whether she noticed large-bodied people, Reiko had been quite adamant she didn't really notice *futotteru* (fat) people and that she certainly didn't have anything against them. At that moment, they were driving past a large man who was standing in the road directing traffic. Dressed in navy blue overalls and boots, the overalls made his stomach protrude in an obvious way.

This seemed to jog Reiko's memory. She began to recount a story in detail about a typically hot and humid summer day at her work in an educational administration office. She had looked up from her computer to find a different man standing in front of her desk. Her office was pleasantly air conditioned, and the hallway he had been waiting in was not, so he seemed to be there simply to enjoy the cooler air. She described him as a large man – larger, she noted, than the road worker they had just passed. "He was dripping with sweat and just standing there," she said in disgust-tinged recollection. Reiko then admitted that what she had told Cindi in the formal interview – that futotteru people didn't bother her – actually wasn't true. That man in her office had really bothered her, and it was simply because he was futotteru (and sweaty). She didn't want him anywhere near her, she now remembered.

These two events that took place thirty years apart in Osaka reflect a complex grappling with what it means to be fat. They tap into deep concerns Osakan people (and Japanese people more generally) share about *futotteru hito*, "fat people." They also highlight that women and men talk differently about bodies, and that age and one's own body size also influence these discourses.

Over the course of a summer, Cindi talked to eighteen Japanese people who all lived in the bedroom communities around Osaka, maintaining what is locally considered a typical middle-class Osakan life. Three of the four men and twelve of the fourteen women were married; the three unmarried individuals all lived for most of their lives with their natal families. Gendered expectations within the context of a household with a married couple at its center thus formed the backdrop for many of their conversations about weight, lifestyle, and responsibility. The fundamental theme across all conversations, however, is that in Japan, for most ordinary folks, being futotteru is a very bad thing.

KUIDAORE OSAKA: THE CITY OF WALKING AND EATING

Osaka is located in the western part of the modern, wealthy, maritime nation of Japan. Osaka is often referenced as the gastronomic center of the country, full of fresh, innovative, wonderful foods and people who love to eat them. There are many delicious treats that define contemporary Osakan cuisine for the denizens of the city, treats like *okonomiyaki*, a cabbage-and-meat-filled wheat pancake, and *takoyaki*, a dough ball filled with octopus meat. Osaka is described as *kuidaore*, "a place where one is prone to become financially ruined due to overindulgence in delicious food and drink."[1]

The reasons for Osaka's gourmand reputation are often attributed, correctly or not, to the proximate inland city of Kyoto, which was the location of the Japanese imperial court from the mid-700s to 1868. An array of desirable goods, including fruits, salt, and imported goods like spices, flowed through the Osaka port en route to feed the imperial court and its attendants.[2] This made Osaka and its port an important part of the Japanese world at that time: *tenka no daidokoro*, the "nation's kitchen."

In 1868, the imperial family relocated to eastern Japan in present-day Tokyo, but Osaka's reputation as the food capital of Japan endures. Today, much of Osaka looks squarely middle class, and, certainly the fourteen women and four men that Cindi interviewed for this book fit easily into this category. The neighborhoods around the busy core are densely populated bedroom communities of tidy dwellings: condominiums and single-family homes often have separate bedrooms for each child, a small parking space for the family car, and a balcony or garden area to hang washed laundry. There are well-kept parks and children's play areas within walking distance. In large condo communities, residents have their own small park or playground on the property.

Walking the streets of suburban Osaka, one sees children outside playing together and bicycles whizzing by. People don't drive much. They say it is so difficult to find a parking spot and that during the long weekday morning and evening commutes, driving a personal car is slow and tedious. It is also costly, given the taxes levied on cars and roadways. It's easier to use the train lines that spread in every direction and the clean buses that make connections to trains easy and efficient, or to walk to where one needs to go. Indeed, the average Japanese adult walks roughly 7,000 steps per day – the equivalent of 3.5 miles[3] – which is 40 per cent more than the average person in the United States walks but a little less than the Swiss.[4]

Every morning and evening, multitudes of school-aged children and business-suit-clad men and women crowd onto buses and trains, standing room only, to commute to work and school. One day during her fieldwork, Cindi encountered a group of women proudly (and overtly) eschewing the train's safety straps and poles, instead relying on their "core strength" to stay upright in the fast-moving commuter train. Cindi saw one of them pat her lower stomach and then over-heard her tell one of her traveling companions: "If I don't hold the strap or lean on the pole, I have to engage my core muscles to stay bal-anced, which is great exercise." While it is not clear how many people think of the train as providing exercise, the trains do reinforce percep-tions about what is a normal size: not only do cushioned seats have pre-formed narrow dividers that can't accommodate wider-framed hips or larger bodies, above the seats there is often a sign indicating how many people should fit in the space. They aren't designed to help anyone large feel that they fit in.[5]

Train stations aren't just a place people walk to and from as they commute to school and work. They are an amazing destination in their own right. One of the largest and most overwhelming is Umeda/Osaka station in the center of the city. Millions (8.2 million) pass through Umeda each day,[6] transferring train lines or meeting up with friends.

Above the station are massive high-rise department stores with whole floors devoted to food, and a massive array of high-end goods to buy. Underground, the station has a vast warren of arcades, lined with thousands of small restaurants. There are dozens upon dozens of affordable options of every type of Japanese cuisine, as well as a global array of additional meal choices (Italian, anyone? How about Brazilian?), and many different snack treats, including the sweet cream and custard filled puffs at Beard Papa and the steamed buns and dumplings at Horai 551. There is, in fact, a whole city under the station, with doctors' offices, bookshops, and boutiques – but most of the thousands upon thousands of small shop fronts are focused on offering delicious food. Indeed, just outside the ticket wickets of the Umeda/Osaka lines are thousands of small eateries, bars, bakeries, and cafés. Here, like at many stations in Osaka, less processed food can be purchased as well: neighborhood green grocers, fruit stands, fish mongers, and sake and rice stores. Nonetheless, every year, more and more of the options for food purchasing in Osaka are prepared and affordable food for people to grab on the way to somewhere else.

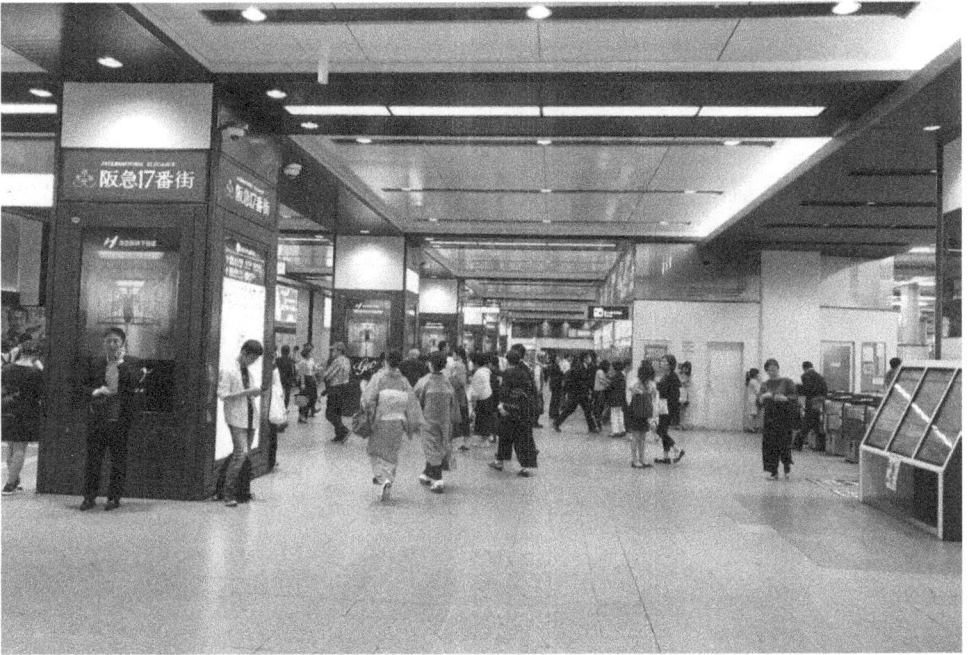

Figure 3.1. The Umeda train station

In Japan, eating out at restaurants has come to be a normal, if not essential, part of everyday life. In contrast to many other countries, relatively more of the population of Japan can afford to eat out regularly because it is a society with a much larger middle class. Eating out has also become cheaper over the years, because of increased portion size, so it makes good economic sense. For a Japanese noodle restaurant (rāmen), the "set meal" (e.g., meal deal) often consists of a steaming bowl of rāmen noodles accompanied by five pot-stickers (Chinese-style dumplings filled with pork), for 900 to 1,200 yen (about US$9–$12), where a bowl of rice (with unlimited refills) can be added for only 100 yen (about US$1).

If Osakans are eating more food outside the home, they are also eating an increasing diversity of food. Much of what is available is more highly processed and higher in oils and fats than what is found in traditional Japanese cuisine.[7] McDonald's, Kentucky Fried Chicken, Shakey's Pizza, German-style beer houses, and Starbucks are now ubiquitous. New and old forms of Japanese fast food[8] restaurants are

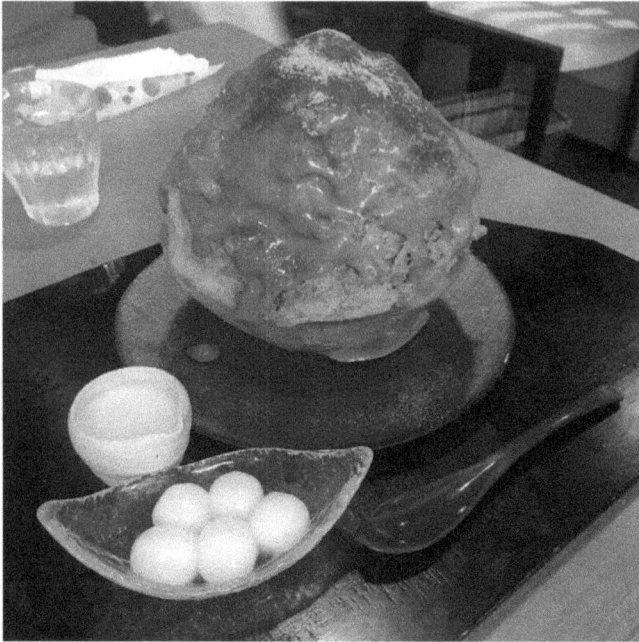

Figure 3.2. Shaved ice with *matcha* (green tea) syrup served with *mochi* and sweetened condensed milk (in pitcher)

nestled alongside these Western establishments. The result is an almost endless choice of conveyor belt sushi, noodles, beef over rice, Japanese curry, European pastries, fries, and burgers.

OBESOGENIC OSAKA AND THE IMPLEMENTATION OF *METABO*

In recent years, the Japanese foodscape has become increasingly obesogenic, meaning it is now an environment that encourages the constant consumption of fattening foods. So, while obesity rates for the country are still low – commonly measured by international and national public health entities all over the world as the number of people with a BMI of over thirty – average adult weights are creeping up. The number of Osakans who are Overweight – once again based on statistical measurements, this time using a BMI of over twenty-five – is low but growing.[9] Importantly, too, scientific studies have shown

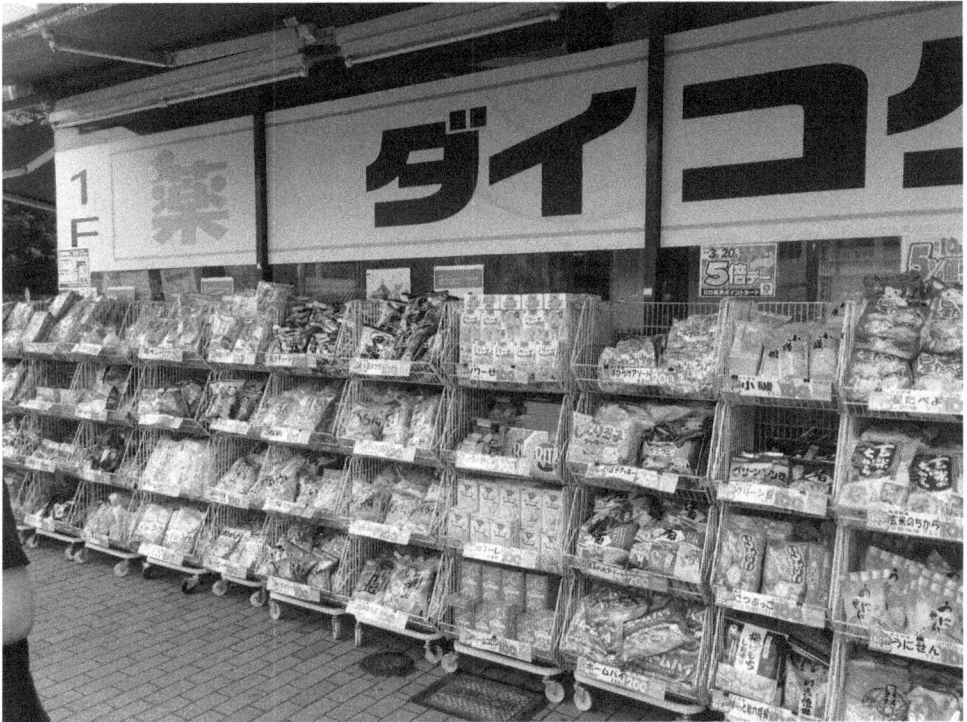

Figure 3.3. Snack foods for sale outside a sundries shop

that metabolic risks associated with weight occur at lower levels of body fat in Japanese people compared to other populations and this research has been widely disseminated in-country.[10] In 2006, Japanese health officials concluded that there was enough evidence indicating that Japanese illness associated with weight was evident at lower body fat levels than in other populations, so they redefined obesity as starting at a BMI of twenty-five.[11] Using this lower cutoff, current Japanese obesity rates jumped from around 3.5 per cent to 32.2 per cent for men and to 21.9 per cent for women.[12]

After lowering the Obesity cutoff criteria and seeing a subsequent dramatic increase in Obese Japanese, the Japanese government declared a national crisis. Obesity was attributed to "the combination of fat eating and lack of physical activity … and the adoption of the Western eating habit."[13] With a low birth rate and a population that leans heavily toward adults and the elderly, the Japanese government is most concerned with the increase of *seijinbyō,* or "adult diseases," including health conditions such as diabetes, hypertension, and coronary disease. In the 1998–9 Annual Report on Health Welfare, the combination of weight gain and diabetes was identified as a serious health problem in Japan.[14]

Other steps were taken to encourage a slimmer Japanese body. Parliament established a Food Education Basic Law (*shokuiku kihon hō*), which aimed to "integrate nutrition advice, agricultural aims, cultural promotion and the engagement of the Japanese public in a single campaign."[15] The law mandated metabolic syndrome health checkups (*metabo kenshin*) for all adult citizens. These checkups have had far-reaching effects on the people with whom Cindi spoke. Thirty-nine-year-old Koichi, for example, patted his stomach as he explained that his company's yearly health checkup entailed measuring the waist and blood pressure of each employee as well as weighing them. This *metaborikku shōkōkun kenkō shinsa* – *metabo kensa* or *metabo* for short – which was enacted in 2008, affects men and women alike. It is an annual mandatory health checkup for all insured citizens between forty and seventy-four years of age in which their abdomens and hips are measured among other metabolic tests.[16]

The health checkup screens are for metabolic syndrome, *not* obesity per se, but obesity is perceived to be an outward indicator of a risky internal state. In particular, a thick waist is taken to be an indicator of either having or being at risk for metabolic syndrome. People with whom Cindi spoke often poked fun at the government's focus on weight, but they also described the lengths that they would go to in terms of calorie counting and exercise prior to the yearly checkup to rapidly lose weight in order to pass the health exam. After the exam, they said, they would return to their previous habits.

Many businesses have also tried to help the people pass the metabo checkup, not by shortening workdays to reduce stress and late-night dinners, but by purchasing software and other technologies that allow workers to track themselves daily, self-monitoring their exercise, fitness, food intake, weight, and health indicators.[17] The metabo law and all this attendant effort hasn't really helped slow the overall increase in weight in Japan at all, at least among men. From 2000 to 2015, the re-estimated rates of obesity (using the BMI>25 standard) increased among Japanese men, rising from 26.7 per cent to 29.5 per cent. In women, however, obesity rates for that same period fell from 21.5 per cent to 19.5 per cent.

WHY ARE PEOPLE FAT? "IT CAN'T BE HELPED"

Koichi, aged thirty-nine, revealed to Cindi at the beginning of their interview that he had gained about 20 kilograms (44.1 pounds) over the previous twenty years. About half of this was put on after getting married. He said it was easy to explain why. It was personal eating habits, worsened by stress and lack of time. He talked of early morning departures for work, skipping breakfast, and eating lunch at a meat and rice (*donburi*) restaurant near his company. He explained that such a daily life is *shikata ga nai* – it can't be helped. But he also articulated that it was his own fault his waist expanded in response to this hectic lifestyle.

Everyone Cindi interviewed, men and women alike, echoed Koichi. It is the individual's responsibility, they said, to curb their appetite and ultimate caloric intake. Everyone also unanimously agreed that children below the age of high school who became fat do so because of poor parenting.[18] Thus, individual responsibility for one's weight and size begins around the age of fifteen and continues lifelong, eventually expanding to include responsibility for one's children's weight and size.

While the *kojin* (individual) was blamed for his/her own weight/ size without hesitation, when asked what kinds of behaviors individuals exhibited that led to becoming fat, the two most commonly listed reasons were time (not enough) and stress (too much). These were then linked to work (for men), school (for students), and home management (for women). As Hanako (who was thirty-eight), said:

> My husband leaves for work before breakfast and often skips his meals. Then, for lunch he eats out at a nearby shop; he usually eats curry-rice, which lacks vegetables and is very heavy. Also, he can't spend a lot of money on lunch food, so it's important he finds something that is filling but cheap. The

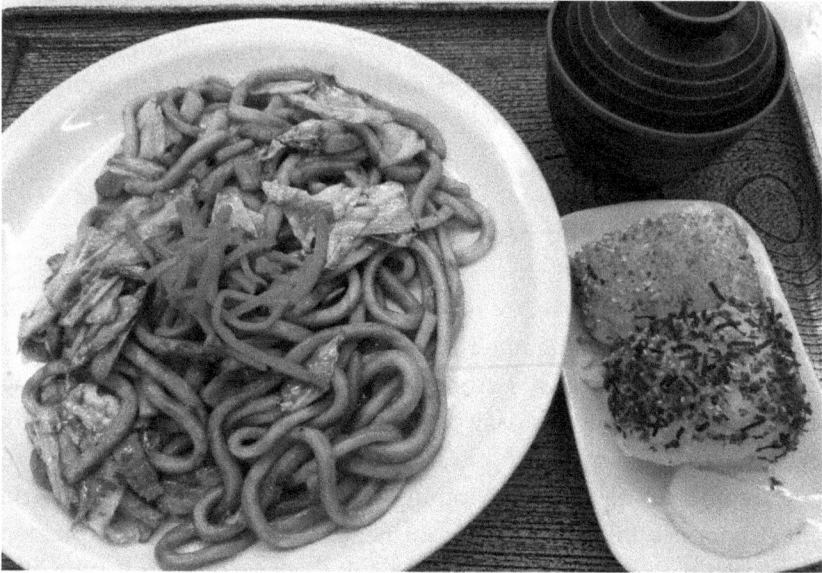

Figure 3.4. A typical lunch "meal deal" of *yakisoba* (fried noodles), *onigiri* (rice balls), and soup

> restaurants near his work are like this [carrying cheap and heavy food] as there are so many company men in that area.

This kind of story was very typical of how married women explained their husbands' increased weights after marriage. All the married women Cindi interviewed reported that their husbands had gained weight after marriage, not because of anything the wives were doing, but because the expectations for work advancement increased, especially after children came along.

For middle-class Japanese families, it is increasingly common for the wife to also work part time, while still taking charge of the household. She is responsible for food acquisition, meal planning, and food preparation. Japanese women – housewives and mothers – thus must bear a double or triple burden when it comes to weight (among other things): they keep track of their own weight, as well as their children's and husbands' weights.[19] When asked about food likes/dislikes, as well as what kinds of foods are healthy and important to eat, the women interviewees answered by speaking for the entire family (not the self), while men answered these questions from the position of the self. Castro-Vázquez refers to this as the "feminisation of care."[20] This is a result of the ways in which gender structures, institutionalized from the early twentieth century on, have placed middle-class women in the role of the manager of the household: taking care of finances, accounting and bill-paying, health and well-being, and scheduler on behalf of all the family members.[21]

For men who work in companies (e.g., *sarariimen*, or salarymen), advancement within the company means longer hours at work (including weekends) as well as more business-related socializing after work. This is typically done over (snack) food and alcohol, which can easily add weight to company workers. Women noted that they, too, gained weight after marriage, but insisted that it was typically put on after having children, especially after the second child. Women's individual weight gain, however, was typically less than their husbands' weight gain, at least according to their own reports. It was husbands who gained the most.

Many of those Cindi interviewed were managing their food intake at the time. At the national level, 50 per cent of young Japanese women report that they have engaged repeatedly and often unsuccessfully in dieting, a direct response to the cultural dictate that women must be slim.[22] This number actually seems low, given the plethora of diet fads and foods/drinks marketed to people in Japan,[23] possibly a result of differing ideas among women about what precisely constitutes a diet.[24] The women Cindi interviewed did not diet per se. Rika, for example, at age twenty-eight, tracked her caloric intake and made a conscious effort not to eat more than she deemed she needed. Kikue (in her early sixties) also spoke of a need to self-police her intake of food – when she had the time. In their own words, Rika, Kikue, and the other women interviewed attributed their weight gain to a lack of "self-time" (*jibun no jikan*). They no longer had time to go to the gym or engage in home exercises, as taking care of (very young) children was time consuming. School-aged children were less time intensive but more expensive, leading most women to seek part-time work while their children attended school (e.g., 9 a.m. to 3 p.m. work shifts), a pattern that again reduced self-time.

Sachiko (in her early forties, with four children) described her days working while the children were at school. When the children had appointments scheduled immediately after school/work, she picked up take-out boxed meals for dinner. Similarly, Aya (in her early thirties) struggled to make sure she was preparing fresh meals from scratch, because it signaled that she was a "good wife and wise mother."[25]

Women like Hikari (in her early thirties) explained the importance of watching what you eat. This could be done by refusing snacks or choosing among high-calorie foods/drinks rather than consuming all of them (e.g., drinking wine at dinner but not eating rice). Rice was unhesitatingly described as a food that most clearly caused weight gain. When young children come home hungry from school or sports activities, rice is often the food they are given to fill them up until dinner. Rice is highly valued in Japan for many reasons; indeed, the word for cooked rice is synonymous with meal.[26] People explained how rice in general is highly nutritious for growing bodies and one of the best food resources for active young people. By contrast, consumption of white rice was seen as requiring tight control in an adult woman to prevent her from eating too much and putting on weight. When Cindi has eaten with Japanese families – either in their homes or at restaurants – she has often seen women either declining rice when offered (at home) or not eating it when served (at a restaurant). Men were far more likely to ask for rice and eat it, sometimes requesting a second helping.

Women worried, too, about their husbands. Sachiko and Hanako, who each had three young children, voiced the greatest concerns about their spouses' weight gain. They spoke at length of their husbands' late returns from work, at which point they would have their evening bath and then eat dinner. This could mean that their husbands were eating at 10:30 p.m. or later. After eating, the men went straight to bed. Thus, the idea of eating just before bedtime was seen as a cause of weight gain, but the women felt there were no solutions to mitigate this. The phrase *"shikata ga nai"* or "it can't be helped" often accompanied these laments. For businessmen, this seemed to be a common outcome of the career trajectory. Men who are in *eigyō* (sales) were reported to be the most at risk for (rapid) weight gain, given the nature of the job, which involved interacting frequently with potential customers while trying to sell them their companies' products. The wining and dining of customers, while not nearly as extravagant as that talked about in the late 1980s and early 1990s (before the economic bubble burst), still required meeting over food and drink on a fairly regular basis. These work obligations for men, combined with the sheer length of their workdays spent seated in front of a computer, were seen as the underlying "culture of work" that contributes to fatness among men in Japan.[27]

One interviewee Cindi spoke with was Masa, a man who self-identified as *futorisugi*, "too fat." Masa, who worked at a large hotel chain, was unmarried at fifty years of age. He lived with his eighty-two-year-old mother, who was somewhat homebound, which limited her ability to "manage" her son in the way that most Japanese women are expected to be responsible for their households. She received calorically and nutritionally appropriate meals from a delivery service every day. Masa typically ate the delivery food that his mother didn't consume, supplementing this with various prepared foods he picked up at a grocery or convenience store. He worked early afternoons through to 10:00 p.m. six days a week; this meant he arrived home around 11 p.m. every night. As he explained, this meant his workday was off schedule compared to that of the stereotypical workday. He typically ate bread and milk for breakfast, bought his lunch (usually rice-based) at a convenience store on his way to work, and ate dinner once he returned home. He usually made rice, ate his mother's leftover delivery food, and then added in prepared food. Masa asserted that what he ate (the contents and meal items) was fairly typical of friends his age, but that the time he ate was not typical. He said that eating late at night was not good at all. He told Cindi, "Ideally, it's best to eat breakfast around 7 a.m., lunch around noon, and dinner at 6 p.m. or 7 p.m. Then, it's best to go to bed about three hours after dinner. This is the best way to live. And, it's better for your body."

Masa described himself as an extremely athletic and active child but noted that he was heavier than other kids his age. When he joined the workforce, his weight started creeping steadily upward. As a young man, he regularly went to a fitness club to work out, but in subsequent years, with his work schedule, he felt he had no time, and this drop in activity level impacted his weight. Masa wryly noted that people had many weight-loss suggestions for him,[28] including that he "eat earlier in the day, eat only one helping of rice, and don't eat fried foods in the evening." When asked what kind of foods he tended to eat along with the leftovers from his mother's meal, he said that he liked fried foods and foods higher in fat. Masa thus attributed his high weight to his food choices and the timing of his meals, but thought the latter more important. If he had a career in which he worked more regular hours, then he felt he would be able to eat meals at their proper times. At the same time, however, Masa placed the ultimate blame for his weight on himself. He stated that lack of self-control was a major factor in any one person's struggle with weight. He said that he saw his fondness for fried and fatty foods as a weakness.

Masa's life story reflects much of what Cindi heard from Osaka company men in general, whether they identified as fat or not. Work requirements regulated their waking, eating, and sleeping. For salary-men, work was the number one factor that impacted their ability to eat quality food in appropriate quantities, and work also required them to stay late and go out drinking and snacking. The way that work reg-iments daily life for salarymen is well documented.[29] Indeed, many laments from men about their lives center on the role that work plays in hindering their ability to help with domestic tasks, be instrumental in child rearing, and become more involved in their families – not just on the ways in which it hinders self-care such as fitness.

Men and women alike articulated the need to practice constant vigilance over their personal habits – especially around food – to control their weight. They identify the pressures of modern Japa-nese work- and school-life that precipitate unhealthy eating habits in terms of reliance on premade, packaged foods; having meals occur at odd times of the day (and night); and the need to eat high-fat, alco-hol-accompanied work dinners in restaurants. Thus, weight gain was attributed to a lack of time and to the stress of modern Japanese life, or modern Japanese middle-class, urban life. Yet despite widespread acknowledgment of the macro forces at work, when asked about re-sponsibility, people unanimously stated the same sorts of ideas about individual responsibility, control, and discipline that we see underly-ing problematic conceptions of stigmatized fat in the West. In other words, fat people were blamed and shamed for what was viewed as a profoundly undesired condition.

In Osaka, looking at futotteru through a gendered lens, it is easy to see the ways in which a family's health and weight rests on the shoul-ders of mothers and wives. Both men and women expressed dread and embarrassment at the thought they might become futotteru. Those who were labeled futotteru, however, were quick to assume personal responsibility, saying that their excess weight was their fault. Men, in particular, overwhelmingly asserted that personal eating habits, lack of time, and feelings of stress created an environment wherein their eating habits went awry, but that ultimately, they should still exert control over themselves. They did not, however, claim responsibility for their wives' weights. Women, on the other hand, claimed responsibility for their own weight status, that of their children, and that of their husbands.

WHEN IS FAT BAD? "DRIPPING IN SWEAT"

In Japan, people with large bodies are often viewed as both a nuisance and an annoyance (*mendokusai*) and disgusting. Setsuko, who is thirty-one years old and very slim, explained there was a common association of fat people and an image of *fuketsu-na*. She noted that if fat people did not keep themselves clean and free of sweat, for example, onlookers felt they would be prone to producing an odor. This image of a fat person typically elicited the term fuketsu-na or "unclean, slovenly," which has the same (im)moral overtones as can be found in descriptions of fat people in the United States.[30] When Cindi asked interviewees to describe a person with these fuketsu-na characteristics, the answer was always the same: *"ase wo fukanakute, kami no ke wa dorodoro"* ([someone who] does not wipe their sweat and their hair is dripping [with oil]). When Setsuko talked about people who exhibited fuketsu-na characteristics, she put a finger to her temple-area mimicking the dripping of sweat and/or oil from the hairline. If there was an open seat next to such a person on a crowded train, she explained, she would never consider taking the seat next to him/her.

Masa, the largest of the men Cindi interviewed, seemed to understand this view. He went to great lengths to keep himself sweat-free and clean-smelling. He carried multiple handkerchiefs to wipe his sweat, and he always had a clean shirt in his bag so he could change if he needed to. He kept his hair oil-free and was conscientious of his personal odor. He was highly aware that Japanese people view smelly, sweaty, and fat bodies as unclean and troublesome. Masa blamed himself for not controlling his size, but he could control his odor and his sweat, and so he was rigidly disciplined with respect to these latter characteristics.

Osakans often expressed sympathy for people they encountered whom they categorized as fat. Again and again, Cindi was told that "when seeing someone who is obese in a public place" the first thought that crossed the viewer's mind was "Are they healthy?" or "I wonder if something is going wrong for them?" This is in direct contrast with how people felt when encountering a very thin person; there was unanimous agreement that when seeing someone who was quite thin, the first thought that came to people's minds was *kowai*, or "scary," and *garigari*, or "skin and bones." People said they did not feel concern for the thin person's health and well-being in the same way that they did for those they perceived to be fat.[31] Participant-observation findings parallel the interview data in this regard. In all her years working in Japan, Cindi rarely witnessed a larger-bodied person being stared at or shamed in public (at least not by adults), but she did witness thin people being overtly noticed and even remarked on (typically by young people) on more than one occasion.

Of course, concern for a fat person, while ostensibly kinder than overt shaming, nonetheless sees the fat body as inherently bad. The comments – most notably, "I wonder if something is going wrong for them?" – also illustrate that this "badness" is not just centered on learned ideas of increased medical risk but on the perception that something is awry socially as well. In this regard, the middle-class segments of Osaka society with which Cindi comes into regular contact certainly display fat stigma, albeit rarely overtly expressed. In fact, when Cindi pressed interviewees, focusing specifically on people's recall of their younger days in school, they did admit that they recalled other students being shunned or explicitly made fun of for being larger than average. Everyone agreed adults do not engage in this kind of rude behavior, or, as one person told Cindi, it is done quietly, so that no one really hears it. In other words, fat stigma goes underground among adults. The most obvious place it surfaces, then, is within family settings. The opening vignette, when the father compared his daughter's legs to a daikon, certainly illustrated this, as did the interview with Masa. Masa reported that he routinely heard from his mother that he should lose weight. A few days prior to the interview, in fact, she had said to him, "If someone sticks a pin into you,

you'll explode," implying his large stomach and body was a bomb waiting to go off. Masa consistently self-shamed to Cindi, saying that he was obese and a "fatty" (this word uttered in English); he did not believe himself to be in good health nor was he satisfied with his physical condition.

WHO IS FAT? "JAPAN DOESN'T HAVE FAT PEOPLE LIKE THE US DOES"

Cindi met Tomoko, a twenty-seven-year-old aspiring graphic artist, in a Mister Donut shop on the corner of a busy intersection on the outskirts of Osaka. Tomoko slowly ate donut holes as she and Cindi sipped bottomless cups of coffee. Tomoko did not describe herself as fat, but she specifically pointed out that she had gained significant weight (some 18 kilograms or 40 pounds) after living in France for a year as a high school exchange student.[32] She explained the gain was due to the rich French cream and cheese. Tomoko admitted that her teenage self was embarrassed at how much weight she had gained, and she was humiliated that she had to return to Japan fatter than when she left. Luckily, as she explained it, within six weeks of being home eating her mother's cooking and following typical daily physical activity routines (walking to and from school, walking to the grocery store, etc.), she returned to her previous weight. Tomoko noted that she also had felt fortunate because during those six weeks, she was able to still wear her school uniform and thus could hide some of her weight under the full skirt.

When Cindi met Yusuke, a nineteen-year-old student, he had just returned from spending the year in a rural area of Illinois (United States) as a high school exchange student. He talked about how his home-stay family did not eat vegetables very often, and, when they did, the vegetables tended to be potatoes or corn. He recalled monotonous daily lunches of nachos, hot dogs, or burritos bought at convenience stores. Yusuke gained 20 kilograms (44 pounds) during that time. He admitted he was so embarrassed by his own weight gain that two months prior to his return to Japan he took up running. It worked, and he was able to return home without the feared humiliation of facing family and friends noticeably fatter. Like Tomoko, Yusuke believed weight gain was a problem that the individual had a responsibility to "fix," but that it was especially hard to do this in Western countries like the United States. Cindi often heard *amerika no yō ni futottenai desu ne* or *amerika no yō ni himan na hito wa inai yo*, both of which roughly translate as "Japan doesn't have fat (*futotteru*) or obese (*himan*) people like America does."

While the Japanese viewpoints are technically accurate, they absolutely fail to capture the nuances of what is occurring on the ground in Japan, and the ways in which there are striking parallels in the thinking of people both there and in the United States when it comes to questions of who is fat, why we are fat, is fat bad, and so on. Moreover, a general palliative, "Japan is not a fat country" type of thinking coincided and contradicted the thinking that saw oneself, one's spouse, and other friends and family members as needing to lose weight and being at least a little obese.

When Cindi asked what kinds of people in Japan were fat, she was frequently told that people with health problems or little self-control were fat. And yet, when Cindi asked individual interviewees if they were fat, many replied that they were most likely *chotto himan deshou ka ne*, "I'm a little obese I suppose." Additionally, all of the younger people Cindi interviewed said that they were not satisfied with their bodies' physical condition with regard to weight. Without hesitation and regardless of their actual size, over and over they noted that they could stand to lose a little weight. Sometimes people added that they needed more physical exercise on a regular basis. But, on the whole, more people focused on their diets. For many Japanese people, especially middle-class people in urban settings, deciding who is fat is not simply a matter of finding one's BMI or even one's waist circumference; instead, it is often about how one feels, the ability to conform to a routinized eating schedule and menu, and how one compares to peers.

Within their own networks of family and friends, people were able to identify those they thought were fat. However, as many people explained, if the personality of a friend was *akarui*, "bright/cheerful," and *omoshiroi*, "interesting/funny," then the size of the body was considered less of a social obstacle. Friends rarely commented directly on each other's bodies. Within families, the story was a bit different. All women told stories of being body shamed by brothers, fathers, or husbands. Setsuko explained that her younger brother would tell her *"chotto yasetara kawaikunaru yo"* or "if you lost some weight, you'd be cute." Fat shaming among family members appears common, therefore, especially men shaming women and parents shaming children. The pattern of these small humiliations thus likely helps also to reinforce the rigid Japanese gender and age hierarchies. The shaming itself might be relatively mild and said in jest. But people understand the deeper meaning. Don't be bad and futotteru: be a thin, worthy Japanese citizen.

INTERVIEWING AND EATING IN OSAKA

Asking people to give of their time, often a substantial amount of time, is part and parcel of undertaking an ethnographic approach to research. Honoring the participants' stories and the time they share is one of many ways we meet our ethical commitment to the project at large and to the individuals specifically. In chapter 2 we talked about the nature of interviews that ask explicit questions around body size, fat, and experiences of stigma; there we noted that we approach such conversations carefully and purposefully. From the outset, then, Cindi arranged and scheduled interviews according to the convenience and comfort of the participants – convenience in terms of interview location, day, and time, comfort in terms of whether the participant wanted to have to negotiate the foreignness of Cindi in public settings. This meant that Cindi crisscrossed the greater part of Osaka multiple times on some days depending on where the participants were living and/ or working. Most of the interviews did not involve food but offered the opportunity for food as they overwhelmingly took place in small cafés.

Older women participants often found their homes to be the most convenient *and* most private. Going to cafés, bakeries, or other public spaces can entail negotiating the presence of Cindi who simply by being non-Japanese draws (unwanted) attention. Sitting in public spaces with Cindi, deep in conversation can elicit raised eyebrows from bystanders or interruptions from others as they wonder, in stage whispers, what the Japanese person and the *gaijin* (foreigner) are doing and what language they are using.

Younger participants, on the other hand, typically chose locations that they wanted to go to; for one participant, talking with Cindi was her excuse to meet at a recently opened, hip European-style café in the newly renovated Osaka City station area. For some participants who lived in the more suburban sprawl areas of Osaka, meeting Cindi was a chance to go to the more urban and trendy areas of the city. Young company men could only meet on weekends due to schedules that were packed with work responsibilities. And, older men relied on their wives to arrange the interview day, time, and place. No matter where the interview took place, a beverage was always available. In private spaces (homes and offices), cold Japanese green tea (*ocha*) or the summer staple barley tea (*mugi-cha*) was offered. In cafés, participants and Cindi ordered what suited their palates that day.

The one exception to this typical pattern was an interview that Cindi did after seeing her own family off at the airport to return to the United States. This interview took place in the participant's home which happened to be on the way to/from the airport. The woman, Megumi, who Cindi has known since high school, had prepared an elaborate dinner that included miso soup, egg rolls, green salad, and individual portions of *chirashi-zushi* – a dish that as the name implies is a kind of sushi. It is a "sushi bowl" rather than a rolled or *nigiri* style of sushi. Sushi rice (vinegared rice) is put into a bowl and then topped with a variety of things which may include raw fish, stewed and sliced *shiitake* mushrooms, thinly sliced omelet, or pickled ginger. In this particular case, the main topping was different varieties of delicately sliced *sashimi*, raw fish. The meal felt celebratory, perhaps because Cindi and the participant hadn't reconnected face-to-face in over twenty years. After dinner, small individual pastries were brought out and coffee was brewed. The son and husband retreated to another part of the house while Cindi talked to Megumi and her college-aged daughter. Being allowed into people's homes, being allowed to hear their personal stories and experiences of fat and body size, is a privilege and honor; sharing a meal with them is icing on the (proverbial) cake.

CHAPTER FOUR

Fat in Peri-rural Georgia, USA

In the fall of 2016, Alex and Sarah were invited to Thanksgiving dinner at Alex's in-laws, about an hour north of the huge city of Atlanta. The drive went past the airport and out into what had, until recently, been farmland. Old farms and little churches were interspersed with cookie-cutter housing developments, gas stations, fast food outlets, and strip malls. The freeway was almost deserted, as everyone was home preparing for one of the most important ritual family meals of the year for most people in the United States. Thanksgiving is an occasion that ideally brings together relatives to eat one large meal of turkey, vegetables, and sweet pies. Across the country, each family has their own way of creating that meal.

As they arrived at the gathering, the men were out in the chilly weather in the garage, deep-frying a turkey in a vat of fat set over a burner. In preparing the Thanksgiving dinner, men often take charge of cooking the meat (seen as a more masculine food, and a more masculine task in the United States). That deep-fried turkey got a lot of attention. It was a new technique for the family, tried only for the second year in a row. It was fast, too, people noted: "It only takes forty minutes in the deep frier!" For the traditionalists, there was a second, oven-cooked turkey waiting in the kitchen.

Many of the women were still bustling in the kitchen, adding the finishing touches to the many vegetable side dishes, "fixings" like stuffing, and desserts. Some recipes had come from Facebook or

Pinterest. Most were old family ones. Alex's mother-in-law had made a huge dish of creamed corn ("I used three different types of corn that I'd frozen from fresh back in September … field corn, which is real difficult to find now, sweet corn from round here and sweet corn a friend brought from Kentucky … the field corn makes it creamier"). Close family friends arrived, bringing more home-prepared food. The table started to become filled with pumpkin pie, banana cream pudding, broccoli salad, boiled collard greens, stuffing, and casseroles of soft oven-baked vegetables. There were also gallons of the Southern staple drink of sweet tea on the sideboard, as well as sparkling water. Even the two-year-old had sweet tea in her bottle. Later, the mother of the two-year-old told Sarah that the sweet tea in the bottle was something reserved for special occasions only and one that she allowed at the older generation's insistence, not because she thought it was a good nutritional practice.

Similar pre-emptive awareness and management of potential critique came up at other times over the course of the meal and afternoon. Alex's mother-in-law, for example, pointed out that she had relied on her garden in earlier times for fresh local vegetables but that now she had to rely on a local food network to obtain fresh local produce. The subtext of her discussion was not only the local-rooted identity wrapped up in these food preparations but also the emphasis on healthy practices, even when these are difficult to maintain.

Of the twenty-two people Sarah and Alex interviewed for this project, everyone lived in rural towns or the suburban sprawl located in an arc across the north of the state of Georgia, just above Atlanta. Georgia is within a zone of the United States referred to as the "American South," with its own regional identity and traditions tied to an agricultural past. Participants in this study were mostly women but did include men; they were a range of ages, worked all sorts of different blue- and white-collar jobs, and were married, never married, or divorced.

Discussions like those noted above occurred quite often over the course of fieldwork in northern Georgia, as many locals are accustomed to grappling with the negative perceptions of the South held by outsiders, whether the focus is on health (obesity), food (fried), education (not enough), or "accent" (too much). Another conversation that ensued during the meal preparation is illustrative. A number of the family members and family friends worked or had worked for a multinational company with offices in Atlanta. One family friend said that the company only allowed her to do liaison work in the South and in Utah because those were the only places that would "appreciate my Alabama accent." One of the younger women pointed out that Southern language varieties routinely are associated with being dumb and uneducated.

Few large family meals in this community begin without thanking God that there is food on the table. When all the food was prepared, everyone was asked to bow their heads while the senior man of the family said a prayer before eating. He grew up in the state but slightly further south, and that afternoon, he talked about his youth, recalling how hungry many people were in the face of the cyclical food scarcity that was still common when he was a child. He said this was why he thought it was important to never take food onto your plate you weren't going to eat.

PERI-RURAL GEORGIA: SOME CONTEXT

The state of Georgia sits firmly in the American South, with South Carolina to the northeast, the Atlantic Ocean to the southeast, Florida to the south, Alabama to the west, and Tennessee to the north. Interstate 20 (I-20) runs east-west across the northern quarter of Georgia, from the old city of Augusta on the state line with South Carolina, through the sprawling, ever-growing metropolis of Atlanta, to the state line with Alabama. Sarah and Alex's fieldwork took them everywhere in the peri-urban sprawl that characterizes the communities north of I-20 and that are not part of Atlanta proper. This included historic small towns, homes set within rolling farmland, and those in new commuter bedroom communities that are rapidly spawning along the highways coming out of Atlanta. The economic and cultural impact of Atlanta (and, to a lesser extent, Savannah and Augusta) is felt throughout the region.

Nonetheless, for much of the twentieth century, rural Georgia – and, indeed, many areas of the rural South, especially those in and

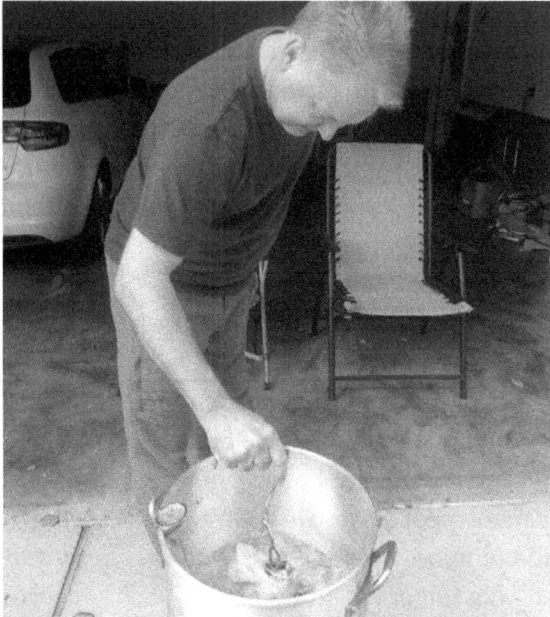

Figure 4.1. A turkey being deep-fried in a garage

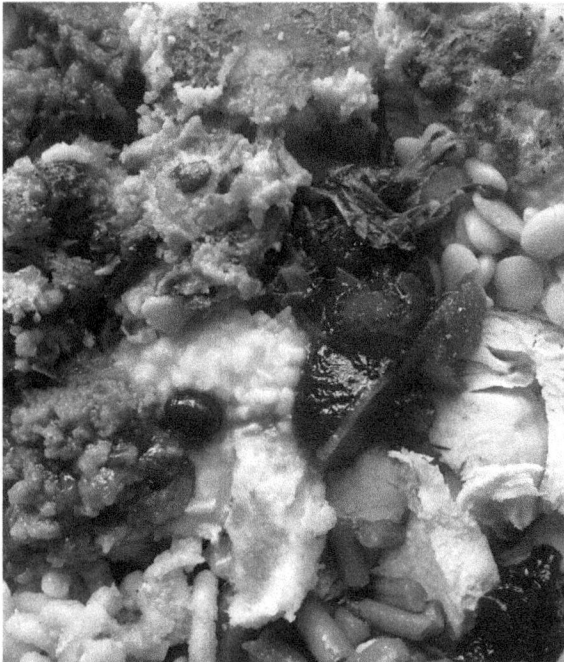

Figure 4.2. A plate at the family Thanksgiving meal

around Appalachia – has been associated in the US imaginary with uneducated, white poverty.[1] In north Georgia, several of the counties in which Sarah and Alex conducted fieldwork sit at the feet of the Appalachian Mountains, a situation that in 2016–17 provided a departure point for urban families vacationing in the national parks, as well as for people interested in exploring the rich tapestry of cultural and economic diversity in the region.[2] Despite such developments, in conversations Sarah and Alex had with locals, the specter of uneducated, ignorant, white poverty still loomed large. One interviewee, for example, said, "You see the guys who run around here in the wife beater T-shirts, and have this rebel flag on the back of their truck, and all that kind of stuff. And it's one of these like, 'I'm going to whip your butt, boy,' kind of thing, you know?"

The counties in northern Georgia where Sarah and Alex worked, talked, and visited with people are predominantly white ones. Atlanta itself is very racially diverse, and some of the planned communities going up along the highways have turned into pockets of racial diversity, but these communities are full of urban professionals oriented around the city. Locally rooted communities are economically impacted by the development and the urban/suburban sprawl, but the cultural exchanges are much more attenuated.

The vast majority of the interviewees were white and, in their discussions with Sarah and Alex about bodies, food, fat, and health, they mostly reflected views that dominate in white sociocultural contexts in the United States. There are, of course, rich discussions taking place in the same region that do not reflect white norms and, in fact, critically engage with them. Sarah and Alex are highly aware, based on these discussions and other research, that race shapes embodied experiences for people in the American South in profound ways. For example, there is a robust literature that delves into body norms and notions of identity among Black women. This literature – and research exploring other communities and racial identities – is important, but not one that the data gathered for this book is able to advance in any meaningful way.[3]

Many people to whom Sarah and Alex spoke grew up in small towns and talked about how much the economics and physical landscape of the area have changed. There are still many old farmhouses standing in fields and overgrown stands of trees in the rural areas, but very few farms are functioning and self-sustaining. The older, small farms that are active raise primarily hay, cows, horses, and a little corn. Another frequent model is a farm/wooded lot that has subcontracted with a well-known national industrial chicken company. The area never had the huge farms that characterize southern Georgia, as it's too hilly and the soil has too much clay. During fieldwork, most people – especially, older people – told Sarah and Alex that locals still have gardens and eat what they grow, but local produce and food products are not a particularly significant source of food for anyone in the surrounding counties. People told Sarah and Alex that poverty is a problem across many of the counties, as is a lack of job opportunities. Many people are unemployed or underemployed. Many of them don't want to move away because they are reluctant to give up their family and other ties to the area: the parents who provide babysitting or a house to share, the relative who has the occasional work opportunity, and so on.

There were Walmarts in most of the strip malls or on the outskirts of the city centers, as well as massive stores like Kroger, Publix, and Petco. The people with whom Sarah and Alex spoke typically shopped at these establishments because they were less expensive and they had a wide range of items available. They tended not to be physically proximate, which necessitated planning regular shopping trips and then driving to them. By contrast, people stopped for fast food after work precisely because the national fast food chains (DQ, Dunkin' Donuts, McDonald's, Chick-fil-A, etc.) could be found in retail strips along the highways and in city centers and they were convenient in addition to being cheap.

Aside from perhaps Chick-fil-A, none of these food purveyors were distinctly Southern. The transformation of much of the urban and suburban landscape in the United States into an "obesogenic (obesity-producing) environment," characterized by many opportunities to eat fast foods, pre-made high-fat/sugar foods, or highly processed foods, as well as by few opportunities to actively move around, has been extensively documented.[4] Also important in this research context – although again, not unique – is that, in part because of the pattern of leapfrog development, there were few alternatives to the big retail chains and it was very difficult to get around on foot (i.e., without a car). There were virtually no sidewalks anywhere Sarah and Alex went, whether one looked along the country roads, in the strip malls, or in the little towns sprinkled throughout, and Sarah and Alex

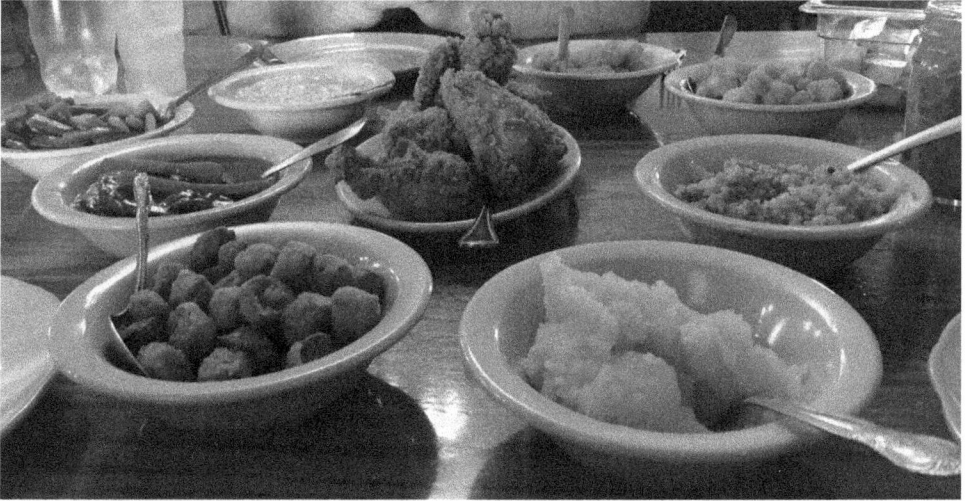

Figure 4.3. Self-consciously Southern: Restaurant versions of regional cuisine

saw few pedestrians or cyclists. The exceptions were the towns that had college and university campuses.

WHY ARE PEOPLE FAT? "ULTIMATELY IT'S OUR FAULT"

In one small town, Sarah stopped briefly at a beautiful little library, and ended up chatting with several of the women there. They reiterated verbally some of the same themes that were so apparent in the local landscape: (1) mixed feelings about the profound changes in the physical landscape wrought by development in recent years; (2) concerns over health; and (3) ambivalence over what exactly constitutes Southern identity. One local remarked that it pained her to see the Atlanta sprawl creeping northward, spoiling all the countryside, but she understood people selling their family acres, because there wasn't much farming or industry in the area to fall back on. An older woman (a recent transplant from New England) chimed in at this point and said that everyone would be healthier if they just followed a Paleo diet. Among other comments, the Paleo dieter remarked, "People 'round here are just not interested in nutrition," and finished with, "Everyone in this country is dying in front of their TVs!"

The overtly stigmatizing, shaming comments about locals and local cuisine effectively shut down the conversation. That said, this woman is not alone in her views about both people in the United States in general and Southerners in particular, and that is an interesting and relevant point.

While visiting a farmer's market in Gainesville, Georgia, for example, Sarah struck up conversations with a couple of local farmers. Most of the farmers were over the age of sixty. One exception was a young local hog farmer who reared only pasture/woods-raised pigs simply because he lost his stomach for the feedlot style of raising. Another exception was a farmer who had actually been born and raised in Atlanta but had moved out to the country ten years previously specifically to run a small, pesticide-free farm. He remarked that the minute he started describing the hard, physical labor involved in helping on the farm, the young local men weren't interested in working for him – "all these men who are younger than I am can't imagine themselves digging a ditch, they just want to sit around on their asses" was how he put it.

Again, in this narrative, we see the specter of the ignorant, unhealthy Southerner making an appearance – at the same time that the narrative also acknowledges profound structural and development-driven change, systemic localized poverty, and deep nostalgia for certain aspects of Southern identity and ways of life. What is striking about these themes that arose again and again in fieldwork is that people relate to them in ways that are deeply complex. One young interviewee (in her early twenties) named Christina, for example, remarked that she didn't feel Southern, but then back-pedaled slightly and said, "I guess I would characterize it as there's definitely a specific way of speaking that outs us as Southerners. I would say politeness is very characteristic of Southern people ... A lot of people would characterize the South as a very hateful, uneducated place ... but I don't think that that characterizes the whole South." Similarly, Anna (in her mid-twenties), was quite critical of her town and, indeed, the South more generally at different points in her conversation with Sarah, but then commented, "I think it's easy for other places to just kind of pigeon-hole the

South … It's okay, you can discriminate against Southerners because they speak that way, they're ignorant. I think that is still such a common stereotype that is out there."

Ultimately, everyone Sarah and Alex interviewed got themselves hung up on the essential question that Sarah and Alex hear repeatedly in their US-based fat and obesity research: whose responsibility is it when an individual/family/community/country gets fat? Sarah and Alex have written about this contradiction elsewhere,[5] but it remains a fascinating one, because the mutually contradictory explanations are so deeply embedded in the national worldview. Mainstream US culture famously prioritizes individual hard work and productivity, as well as self-improvement projects and personal responsibility, and these values get applied to fat bodies and soaring national obesity rates (i.e., explanations in the United States for *why we get fat* come back again and again to notions of personal irresponsibility, lack of knowledge and effort, and even laziness).[6] Medical admonitions to lose weight, vocal public health programs, and a vast diet and exercise industry reinforce these ideas with their emphasis on changing people, not policies.

Despite this overwhelming set of cultural beliefs, most people in the United States have been exposed to enough public health messaging about obesity that they also have absorbed basic facts such as (1) Obesity rates have dramatically increased in the United States recently because of increased availability of fast food, packaged food, and high-fat/high-sugar foods and (2) poverty increases your risk of being Obese. Indeed, much of the *official* public health messaging about Obesity rates in the South has focused on these two explanations for why the region shows higher rates of clinical Obesity and Overweight, even compared to the rest of the country. *Cultural* explanations in the United States, however, return again and again to notions of laziness, ignorance, and irresponsibility. In north Georgia, these explanations are amplified by lingering stigma attached to Southern identity and, in particular, to poor white Southern identity.

The interview data shows people pulling from two very different explanatory models to explain why people in (1) Georgia, (2) the South, and (3) the United States more generally are fat. On the one hand, interviewees clearly cited structural and political economic causes underlying obesity. Amy (in her late twenties) had a characteristic analysis, saying,

> With the 1950s, you start to see frozen foods come out and TV dinners ... and, of course, as time goes on, you have more women working outside the home, and you have parents having to give their kids the key to the house so they can let themselves in after school ... And I think, in the South – I've seen some kind of articles and food studies like this – where you have higher instances of poverty, you have more proliferation of fast food restaurants and fewer health options for food. And this is a poor area.

Christina said something very similar, commenting,

> I mean, I'd like for everybody to look healthy and have a healthy lifestyle. But I think with a lot of the wealth distribution it's just not something that's possible. Because a lot of these people are working very low-income jobs or not working at all and then they have kids ... With just like the diet, the processed foods that obviously weren't around ... I think now obesity is way more common.

Both women, in other words, cited large-scale economic and social factors in their responses at this point in their narratives. Caroline (in her early fifties) echoed these same themes of massive structural and environmental change over time, combined with wealth and privilege (or lack thereof), influencing fatness and weight. She said,

> Back when I was growing up, they didn't have all the GMOs and the horrible things in the food ... You're gonna spend more money to eat healthy ... So it's very hard to eat healthy anymore ... If you have the income, you can do just about anything. Especially eating healthy, being able to afford a gym membership.

Caroline spoke from the perspective of someone who could not afford a gym membership and struggled to buy healthy food, while working for wealthier people. She saw stark economic contrasts every day.

Anna and Kevin picked up these same themes in their interviews, but also discussed them in the context of the local foodscape, "Southern cooking," and localized eating habits. Anna described watching the young people in her town invariably head straight to the frozen food aisle at the supermarket (in contrast to older folks, who bought staples), but then said,

> And I know part of that is they're probably working a terrible job, and they don't have a lot of money, and they probably don't have a lot of time. So, they need something that's quick that doesn't require any prep work. But I also think they probably grew up eating a lot of that, because their parents were in that situation.

Anna highlighted that poverty inhibits what one can buy in today's landscape, but also said that people nowadays have lost their connection to the land and healthy eating habits. In her interview, she contrasted the current pattern with the lifestyle of her grandparents, who had very little money but were self-sufficient and relied on what they and their neighbors grew. Kevin (in his early sixties) told a story from when he was young, when he visited a friend, Henry, who lived in a rural area further south. He described massive meals at his friend's grandmother's farmhouse, saying

> And of course the food was groaning, we were bending the tables ... it was that sort of country cooking ... Anyway, I'm sitting next to Henry's mama, and she pulls out this, like, double caramel chocolate butter nut coconut cake. And she says, "Henry, how about some cake?" And he says, "Mother, I can't, I'm just too full." I'm like, "Thank God, I can refuse now," because I was about to pop. "Henry, I spent two hours baking this cake, and you're going to have some." So, she got to me. "Yeah, just a little slice please." Plop, plop, you know, about a third of the cake.

Kevin went on to underline the fact that a groaning table and a Bible-sized slice of cake weren't necessarily a problem for Henry's grandmother or parents because of all the physical labor that accompanied their eating. In Kevin's view, the problems arose for his and

Henry's generation. Kevin went on to point out that people today still want to eat butter, lard, oil, and sugar, but that they no longer labor for it in the same literal sense of generations past. He very clearly included himself in this pattern and had a number of unflattering observations about himself.

Many other interviewees, especially the younger ones, noted that the stereotype of Southern cooking was based on fried, heavy food. The younger ones tended to be rather dismissive of relying on such cooking because of its perceived negative impacts in terms of weight and health. Others had a more complicated view. Charlene (in her late thirties), for instance, said,

> I think that's the way Southern food is, it kind of sounds ridiculous, but emotions [are] in food ... That people care about what they make and what they serve to others ... But it's hard to cook traditional Southern food and still try to stay healthy. And my husband and I, you know, the older you get, the harder it is to maintain a healthy weight. So, we don't cook Southern food a lot ... Because when I was growing up, this is all I ate. And I see the product in my parents ... Well, my mother is a diabetic, high blood pressure.

For Charlene, Southern cooking was about love and connection and nostalgia. Yet she avoided it because she drew a direct connection between ill health and fat and eating Southern cooking.

Anna bluntly pointed out, "I don't see a lot of people cooking those [traditional Southern] foods ... what I see mostly is, you know, the Chick-fil-A backed up, or the McDonald's." Anna echoed what many older interviewees who grew up with large gardens and farms told us: weights went up when processed food consumption went up, and blaming Southern cooking for local weight gains blames traditional culture when the blame should rest on infrastructure change and individuals' *loss* of traditional ways. As Anna observed, people know how to drive to Chick-fil-A but they no longer know how to "cook from nothing."

Implicit in this critique is the notion of personal responsibility as an explanation for why people gain weight and get fat. Even as people talked about the overwhelming structural, environmental, and economic drivers of Obesity rates in the United States, they kept returning to the idea that people still have the power to make choices and to the idea that people in the United States more generally and Southerners in particular are choosing poorly when it comes to their health. We see this surfacing in Anna's comments about what people buy in the grocery store and Kevin's reference to people wanting to eat fatty, sugary foods even though they no longer work for them.

Interviewees were even more vehement that health and weight are a personal responsibility when they talked about themselves, their family, and close friends or colleagues. Kevin, for example, talked about his own struggles with weight and was quite forthright about just how difficult these struggles had been. He then said, "And you know, I recognize that I can't be a victim here because I could stop … I look at somebody … who's lost a lot of weight … [who']s been disciplined about it … that can be a little painful, because 'Well, why can't I be that disciplined?'" Caroline said markedly similar things in her interview. She stated,

> Looking at me, you wouldn't know I'm a health-conscious person because I *am* pretty healthy *[laughs]*, but I am really actually very health conscious … I mean, all I'd have to do is just work out and eat right. Just, you know, it's called discipline … Yeah, I know what to do. I just don't do it right.

Elsewhere in the interview, Caroline mentioned that she was very overweight and that was the subtext to her comment that "you wouldn't know I'm a health-conscious person." This was also the reason why her narrative sounded rather contradictory: she said first that she was healthy, then that she didn't look it, and then that she needed to be more disciplined and was highly aware of what was "right." By this, she meant that she was already pretty healthy but that to lose weight, she needed to be more disciplined.

Self-control, self-discipline, responsible choices: these were all powerful themes that ran throughout the interviews. Interviewees could and did articulate very informed positions about food deserts, transitions in lifeways and eating habits over time, and the structural effects of poverty and exclusion. Some interviewees even talked extensively about the ways in which the government was failing/poisoning its people through its emphasis on agribusiness and policies that produced food that couldn't be trusted and wasn't "real food." Yet, whenever Sarah and Alex asked, interviewees retrenched back to the idea that if an individual really was committed to health, that individual could be healthy, regardless of context. In this, interviews tapped into cultural frames of reference that are core to the United States, not ones that are specifically Southern.

WHEN IS FAT BAD? "FAT IS ALMOST ALWAYS BAD (BUT BE CAREFUL WHO YOU SAY THAT TO)"

The people with whom Sarah and Alex spoke and interacted in peri-urban north Georgia mostly adhered to mainstream US views that fat is bad, although fat meant different things to different people. Fat, in other words, was a vague description that could encompass a spectrum of higher body weights. Although most people felt that being fat was never good, many also pointed out that an individual could be a bit fat without being diseased and disgusting.

In contrast, most people Sarah and Alex interviewed drew a direct correlation between Obesity and disease, reflecting a feeling that Obesity was a serious, medicalized state. Charlene, in the preceding section, pointed out that her own mother had diabetes and high blood pressure. Most interviewees mentioned these, along with heart disease, as being associated with Obesity specifically. Amy, for example, said:

> I think of ill health, in this respect, as being Obesity rates. I personally am bigger than I would like to be. I would like to lose more weight ... I would be healthier if I made better food choices. And, in my mind, healthier is always less weight ... I'm afraid of developing diabetes ... from seeing my father's side of the family struggle with obesity, diabetes, and high blood pressure.

Anna reflected similar themes, talking first about how she herself used her weight to gauge how healthy she felt physically and then contextualizing this with a story about her mother:

> My mom is a prime example. Heart disease, she had a stroke at the age of sixty ... It is what it is. But diabetes, you know?

> She has lost vision completely in one eye, and she's lost all peripheral vision in the other eye ... That is due to the way that she eats. She eats a certain way, and she doesn't really care for herself in the way that she should with the diabetes. And since she's not eating the way that she should, the weight goes up.

Interviewees – especially those who were older, had relatives suffering from chronic illnesses, or who were not entirely satisfied with their current weights – tended to portray Obesity as being diseased. Some, like Amy in the narrative above, also drew connections between simply being bigger and having an elevated risk for diabetes, high blood pressure, and the like.

A subset of the interviewees – all under twenty-five, female, thin, fit, and active on social media – did critique the "pathologization" of Obesity in the United States to some extent. Christina was very characteristic in this regard. She said: "I've definitely gotten way better about my idea of other people's bodies ... I've had a lot of people that I would classify as really fat beat me like up a mountain and not be out of breath at all. And their skin is glowing, and they look great, so I just am like, 'Okay.'" Here, Christina highlighted the fact that to be fat is not necessarily to be unhealthy, and she pointed out that she came to this conclusion only recently. She then went on to talk about the fact that fat is often viewed as socially bad in the United States, and that this, too, needs to be critiqued. She described the progress that fat activism and size acceptance movements have made at a national level and then talked about the impact these have had on her friends, particularly through social media. Her conclusion was that the online discourse and activism has significantly impacted the ways in which the women of her generation view bodies. She also noted that there was a feminist angle to the movement (although importantly, she did *not* use the word "feminist" herself).[7] Another significant thread for Christina was that her family, although fat themselves, stigmatized fat all the time. She remarked,

> I was raised very much under the impression that fat people are now an abomination. Like they need to be shamed. And that's not at all my way of thinking now ... Cuz again, my

> whole family is pretty fat. So I think it's this hatred of the self
> but projected onto other people ... The impression is they're
> lazy. They eat off of welfare. They don't do anything. Like fat
> people are equated with bad people.

Shame and blame, assumed moral turpitude and lack of discipline, and a reading of the outward body as symbolic of being out of control and a burden are all classic components of fat stigma as it is felt in the modern United States.[8]

Interviewees in Georgia related many stories in which fat was read as socially bad by family members, potential romantic partners, friends, and workplace colleagues and superiors. Charlene, for example, said,

> I've got a couple of friends, and they are extremely over-
> weight. And my first impression is sloppy. And I mean, they're
> nice people. And I hate that that's the first thing that I think
> about. And I just think my high and mighty stance of, "Well,
> why are you drinking a Dr. Pepper every day? Why are you
> drinking five a day?" [is unkind] ... But yeah, the first thing
> is they just look sloppy. And they may not be. They could be
> dressed fine.

Charlene explicitly mentioned that fat for her looked sloppy, but implicit in what she said was that fat also means undisciplined and irresponsible consumption. Other interviewees talked extensively about the ways in which fat stigma influenced their ability to be successful at work, especially when it was associated with a Southern language variety.

Most interviewees were very firm that gender had a profound impact on bodies and on the ways in which body size and eating habits were interpreted and judged by others. Kevin, for instance, despite his own negative experiences with his weight, said that he felt the social and work consequences for women of larger frames were far worse than they were for men. Anna agreed, saying:

> I think, honestly, if you are a white male ... a more well-off
> white male, you seem to fit in ... When people say, "Oh, he's
> a big guy," they think big and strong. But what they actually

mean is, "No, he is overweight. He is a large, massive human."
But it's okay to be that way if you're a big guy – a white male.
You can throw your weight around, metaphorically, but also
literally.

Many women we interviewed voiced this sense that while national masculine body ideals put pressure on men to achieve a toned, not-fat body, local ideals that a man must be big, strong, and protective did give men more leeway when it came to how large size/heavier weight was "read" socially. Women, by contrast, usually reported feeling that they either needed to be petite, looking in need of protection, or at least tiny at the waist. Caroline remarked, "Women should be perfect and men aren't perfect [and don't have to be] … Most women's expectations of men are very, very low. If they can get a few good attributes [in a man], they're doing good."

In fact, gender, in the context of weight, turned out to be one of the most heated topics across interviews. Many (though not all) of the women interviewed became quite upset, discussing the lived inequalities they had experienced or witnessed in terms of the differential pressures put on women versus men to maintain a certain look and weight. This also turned into an avenue for discussing Southern-ness, and what a Southern woman or man was supposed to look like. Amy reported:

Fat was the scary thing that happens to girls, and they
shouldn't be or else they'll never get boyfriends … Even
though the general population doesn't fit that size, that's
still the projected … idea of what the American woman is.
Especially in Southern culture, I think there's still that focus
on traditional femininity … And petiteness is a part of that
traditional femininity … With a [fat] girl, that's breaking away
from that feminine ideal … and, unfortunately, the stereotype is, well, she just lays around all day and eats Cheetos …
Or she's really dumb because somehow, dumb and fat are cor-
related in this stereotype.

Thus, we see that, overwhelmingly, people either tended to view fat as bad and/or they routinely encountered other people who expressed the view that fat is bad. This is not at all surprising, given the extensive research on fat stigma in the United States. People mulled over judgments and stereotypes, their own and others, and in general, were thoughtful across all of these assumptions. Even in the United States, fat is not viewed as always bad, all the time, by all people. It's not even viewed as always bad by the same people at any given time. This, too, shows that people juggle seemingly contradictory models.

WHO IS FAT? AMERICA THE FAT

Again and again, interviewees noted that being in the United States and being Southern increased one's risk of being fat – especially when one lacked financial resources. "America is the fattest country in the entire history of the world" is a common refrain Sarah and Alex heard from people. While not technically true, this certainly sums up what many people believe about residents of the twenty-first-century United States.

As was pointed out earlier in this book, public health initiatives have successfully taught most people that the United States has experienced exponential increases in Obesity across all age cohorts. Everyone Sarah and Alex spoke to in north Georgia referenced some part of these facts and statistics. Amy's comments are illustrative in this sense. She said: "We went from this kinda feast or famine mentality to the dawn of more health conscientiousness … but I don't necessarily know if we're using that information … we know it's bad for us, but are we actually going to act on it?" In this instance, "we" refers to people in the United States as a whole. Amy went on, however, and said that in the South, "We do view food more celebratorially." In this case, the "we" refers to Southerners and echoes comments in earlier sections in which some interviewees perceived the South as having to face particular challenges stemming from the local food landscape. Anna parsed it slightly differently, saying,

> [Thin body ideals are] jammed down our throats from other parts of the country … [but] it's the rural area that incurs that rural poverty, that lack of knowledge, and things like that, that do contribute to being overweight … Maybe that's not true, maybe there's just as high a population of obese people everywhere, I don't know.

Kevin and Patrick both made comments that paralleled Anna's, highlighting both lack of infrastructure and education in rural areas as contributing to overweight. Both men, however, also pointed out that these issues plagued many areas of the Midwest, Northeast, and Northwest – not just the South.

The first overarching conclusion of most participants, therefore, was that weight was a persistent issue plaguing the country as a whole in the twenty-first century. The second overarching conclusion was that problems stemming from both weight and weight-related stigma assumed slightly different forms, depending on region and context. What participants could not agree on, however, was whether the South fared worse in terms of both weight and stigma, compared to the rest of the United States.

INTERVIEWING AND EATING ACROSS GEORGIA

The team said at the outset of this book that in order to produce good data and also meet personal ethical standards around social justice, interviews need to be comfortable for the person being interviewed. This is the first priority – every time Sarah or Alex conducts an interview. Earlier chapters focused on how this priority translates into interview style and content, but it also affects interview setting. All the people interviewed picked the location of where they wanted to be interviewed. For the older folks, this typically meant that Sarah drove to their house and interviewed them in their yard, on their porch, or in their living rooms. Significantly, although everyone interviewed at home offered Sarah something to drink when she arrived, no one felt obligated to feed her – in other words, the visits were not seen as purely social visits (and in contrast to what Jessica describes in her chapter focused on Samoa). Other family members also gave the interview a fair amount of space and privacy – even when both husband and wife were being interviewed, they didn't sit in on each other's interview or eavesdrop.

The vast majority of those interviewed were working full work days or attending some sort of institution of higher education. For some people, this meant that Sarah met them in their office on a break of some kind, and interviewed them there. Often, however, interviewees chose a neutral public place and inevitably, this neutral, public place was a coffee shop of some kind. Coffee shops were a particularly popular choice for those interviewees substantially younger than Sarah herself (possibly, they simply enjoyed the coffee and tea; possibly, Sarah reminded them of a professor or parent and they wanted to talk to her in a more impersonal setting). Iced tea, hot black coffee, and hot lattes were the most popular choices among those interviewed – the only ones who commented on their selection to Sarah ordered unsweetened iced tea and made a point of telling her that they omitted the customary sugar for health reasons.

Sarah ended up drinking coffee at Starbucks (plus, a few independent shops) sprinkled across the arc of northern Georgia in all sorts of weather, recorder parked in front of her on a variety of spindly-legged café tables. Perhaps the two most remarkable interviews took place the day before Hurricane Irma swept into the state. Both young women interviewed on that day declined to postpone their interviews, but the café owners did not feel similarly – all the shops closed prior to the hurricane's arrival. In consequence, each interview took place alone on the porch of the closed down café. By the time of the second interview in the mid-afternoon, the wind was gusting through the streets with considerable force. Listening to the audio recording afterward, one can hear an eerie swooshing noise in the background, behind the two voices, as the wind steadily rises. These two interviewees also had to do the interview without coffee.

CHAPTER FIVE

Gordura (Fat) in Encarnación, Paraguay

Samira bustled around her small kitchen. She was preparing a meal to celebrate the baptism of Amber's youngest son and her godchild in her neighborhood's crowded Catholic Church. It was Sunday morning, and Samira was excited to prepare and serve the beloved dishes that form a typical Sunday meal in Paraguay. The *asado paraguayo* (Paraguayan BBQ), grilled by men, includes ribs (beef or pork), pork sausages, and other meat dishes. The meat is accompanied by side dishes, prepared by women, like *mandioca* (manioc) and *sopa paraguaya* (a juicy cornbread rich with cheese and corn kernels). The savory salad could be simple (cucumbers, carrots, and vinegar) or *ensalada rusa* ("Russian salad," with cooked potatoes, carrots, peas, onions, and mayonnaise). There would be plenty of *gaseosa* (soda pop) and *cerveza* (beer), too.

But this was a special occasion: it was not only the baptism but also a celebration of the much-anticipated annual visit by Amber, her husband, and two young sons.

Samira had asked her husband what dish would make that Sunday meal extra special. Manuel suggested he would drive upriver and bring back a nice, fat fish to throw on the barbeque. In recent years, once-common *dorado* and *surubí* fish[1] had become a rare delicacy in the southern Paraguay city of Encarnación. The Yacyretá Hydroelectric Dam,[2] which straddles the Paraná River between Paraguay and Argentina, had reduced fish populations and fishing grounds. Life had changed in other ways, too. After the Yacyretá Dam flooded Encarnación's beautiful

Paraná River coast, the *encarnacenos* – or "residents," including Samira and Manuel – were relocated, with heavy hearts, to a small piece of land in a resettlement zone at the margins of the city. Unlike their old home, Samira and Manuel now had no family nearby and the neighbors were strangers. There was no space to raise chickens or grow a garden. But Samira and Manuel made the best of it, painstakingly building a new family business: a *tienda*[3] (general store) attached to their home.

Samira glanced proudly at their large, prospering store, pleased that she was sure to have on hand the many special treats her new godson was sure to request. Running the store was tiring – it was practically a 24/7 job – but it allowed her to stay home with her baby. Samira's schedule left little time to exercise and prepare low-calorie meals, and Samira had put on a few kilos since her second child's birth. "Oh well," she joked later to Amber, while they were taking pictures after the baptism celebration: "I'll just stand behind the chair." Samira's body is around average size for a woman her age in the community. From Samira's perspective, gaining a little weight wasn't a big deal, since nobody expects a Paraguayan woman at her age to worry much about her weight anyway.

Amber conducted sixteen formal interviews and two informal interviews (during participant-observation) for this study. The sixteen interviewees were drawn from very different social classes and situations and from neighborhoods in different parts of Encarnación. Eight of the women were married, and the four men were partnered to women in the sample. Of the remaining women, two were divorced; one was an unmarried single mother; and one was unmarried, single, and childless. Even so, many lived in complex extended family arrangements or were intimately involved with their extended family (despite living separately). As such, large and extended families formed the backdrop for many of their conversations about food, fat, and health.

ENCARNACIÓN, PARAGUAY: SOME CONTEXT

Nestled against the Paraná River along Paraguay's southeastern border with Argentina, Encarnación is a small city of around 125,000 people. Known as Paraguay's "Pearl of the South," Encarnación is celebrated for its glorious summers, beautiful beaches, modern board-walk, elegant restaurants and nightlife, and Carnaval festivities. Ask an *encarnaceno* what makes them special, and you'll be told, "*We are gente culta*": cultured people. Encarnacenos pride themselves on being cosmopolitan, well-educated, and open-minded. This pride is on display throughout Encarnación: parks and plazas are well-maintained; city streets are swept clean. It's safe to walk outside or play in city parks well into the night. This cosmopolitanism can also be seen in Encarnación's wide array of international foods and restaurants, and its population's embrace of its many immigrant communities.

The city itself was founded by the Spanish Jesuit priests who ruled Paraguay in the 1600s, and the population remains mostly comprised of people of mixed Spanish and Indigenous Guaraní ancestry. Describing this period, Pope Francis characterized Paraguay's Jesuit missions as "communities which did not know hunger, unemployment, illiteracy or oppression."[4] After Jesuit priests adopted the Indigenous Guaraní as their lingua franca, the Guaraní language flourished, and today up to 90 per cent of Paraguay's mestizo (mixed Indigenous-Spanish heritage) population speaks Guaraní[5] or Jopará (colloquial Guaraní/Spanish mix). The favorite foods of Encarnación and Paraguay – *chipa guasú* ("big" cheesy cornbread), *vorí-vorí* (cornmeal dumpling soup), *mbeyú* (manioc pancake), and *mbaipy-so-ó* (beef and polenta stew) – are generally named in Guaraní and carry the unique flavor of Paraguayan history.

Guaraní myths and legends celebrate cleverness and tricksters, and Paraguayans have long relied on their cunning to make ends meet. After the devastating War of the Triple Alliance in the mid-1800s, Paraguay lost much of its land and 60 per cent of its population. In the years that followed, Paraguayan livelihoods were gutted by rapacious neighboring countries, corrupt dictators, and raw deals with international agencies.[6] The Jesuit era was long over, and hunger became widely known. Internationally, Paraguay developed a reputation for smuggling,[7] arms and narcotics dealers, and other illicit activities. In Encarnación, the import/export economy is a bit more mundane – yerba mate tea, soybeans, beef, and cooking oil are among the goods whose border crossings follow the cadence of international exchange rates. But encarnacenos still proudly tell tales of grandma's adventures of smuggling household goods out of Argentina, across the Paraná River in a reed raft, and into Encarnación's market district.

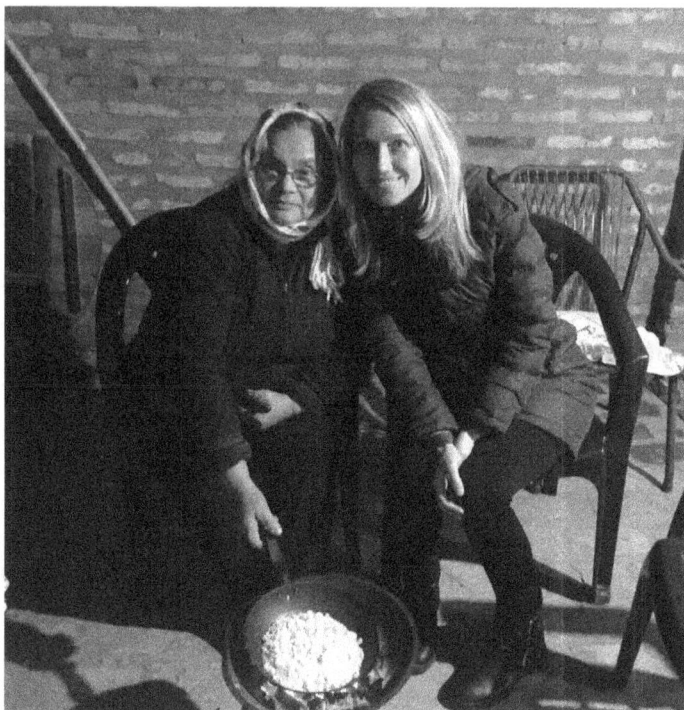

Figure 5.1. Amber enjoying homemade *mbeyú* with Doña Lorenza Avalos on a cold winter night

The planned flooding from the Yacyretá Dam destroyed that historic market district. Authorities promised to invest in economic growth, but the reality of Encarnación's new economy has been mixed. The gorgeous boardwalk and beaches were built, and summer tourists flocked in from all over Paraguay and Argentina. New restaurants, hotels, and other service industries sprung up to accommodate tourists, increasing local employment opportunities. Yet the tourism also brought unwanted cultural changes. Fast food restaurants glutted the city, and many encarnacenos began to incorporate these inexpensive foods in their diets. The pace of life hastened, leaving little time for the social activities that Paraguayans cherish. New sedentary pastimes distracted children from healthy, athletic games they used to enjoy. And many of the promises made to encarnacenos were broken. The resettlement communities were never completed; streets remain in ruins and half-finished parks are padlocked shut. Many families never received their financial settlements. The hoped-for soccer stadium was never built.

Encarnación is a city in economic and cultural transition. These changes reverberate through encarnacenos' pace of life, economic opportunities, daily activities, foodways, and social networks. They are embodied in encarnacenos' weight, their body shapes, and their identities. And they have profound implications for how encarnacenos see themselves and each other.

WHY ARE PEOPLE FAT? "WE EAT BADLY"

In Paraguay, as in many cultures, food is an enormous source of national identity and pride. *Asado* (BBQ) is a common feature in the cuisine of all Southern Cone countries, but Paraguayans can make a strong case that their asado paraguayo is the tastiest. At the heart of Paraguayan cuisine is its breads: sopa paraguaya, chipa guasú, and chipa (made of manioc flour and cheese) are all baked in a traditional Paraguayan outdoor oven called a *tatakua*. As Paraguayans will readily admit, most of these beloved dishes are calorie dense. Antonia, a fifty-two-year-old housewife who worked part-time as a cleaning woman, explained to Amber: "We eat badly in Paraguay, that's why we have obesity, and that brings us diseases. It's the traditional food. For example, *reviro* [a dough made from flour and fat], *tortilla* [frybread], *sopa*. This needs to change."

To manage the heaviness of a traditional Paraguayan diet, people have developed a consensus about the rhythms of daily and weekly meal consumption. Historically, the ideal diet included breakfast, *tereré rupá* (mid-morning snack) followed by tereré (cold yerba mate tea), a heavy lunch, *merienda* (afternoon snack), and dinner. Over time, people have dropped two, three, or four of these meals, as labor became less physical and caloric needs decreased. For example, Juan (a forty-nine-year-old tailor) recounted how much he had eaten in the old days, and then concluded that nowadays, "I have *café con leche*, sweet bread for breakfast, stew for lunch ... and dinner: *café con leche* again, just something light."

Beyond this, there is a widely agreed on weekly menu. The first time Amber tried unsuccessfully to get her favorite Paraguayan meal – vorí-vorí (cornmeal dumpling soup) – on the wrong day, she was surprised to learn that it wasn't just households that adhere to the weekly menu, but that restaurants follow it too. Neider, a thirty-seven-year-old woman who sells clothes in the newly constructed market, described how her family adheres to Paraguay's weekly food rhythms:

> Monday would be soup, that's traditional: *poroto* [bean soup] or *locro* [hominy and meat soup]. Then Tuesday is *guisito* [stew], maybe stew with rice or noodles. Wednesday, for example, can vary. We'll mix it up: if Tuesday was beef, we'll have chicken on Wednesday. It could be baked chicken with white rice and vegetables or sometimes with *chipa guasú*. Thursday we'll sip a soup, because Friday we'll do something more. For example, a potato *pastelón* [casserole]. Always with salad. Or Fridays could be *milanesa* [breaded fried meat]. Saturday will be pasta. And Sundays: *asado* [BBQ].

The Monday meal, a light soup, is considered particularly essential after the overindulgence that is common on Sundays. "It's a Paraguayan tradition," Neider explains. "I was taught that Monday is always soup because we eat quite a bit of BBQ on Sundays."

Cooking, eating, and drinking are often highly communal events in Paraguay. Many Paraguayan dishes are made over open fires, on outdoor grills, or in large shared ovens, making cooking and baking a group activity. The most important communal event in Paraguayan life, however, is the consumption of tereré (the cold-water version of Argentina's mate). A group of two to twelve people will gather around one *jarra* (water jar), *guampa* (cup, traditionally carved from a bull horn), and *bombilla* (metal spoon). The host pours and passes the cup to each person in turn. This activity can go on for hours, especially in evenings, as people tell stories and jokes and talk about their problems. Children frolic around the grownups. While many societies have seen these kinds of communal activities discarded in favor of television, the internet, and other solitary pastimes, even middle- and upper-class Paraguayans have made a serious effort to preserve these customs. For example, walking along the Paraná River boardwalk most evenings, groups of Paraguayan families and friends can be found sharing tereré on benches or folding chairs – across the street from Encarnación's glitziest restaurants and nightclubs.

While nearly everyone Amber interviewed described traditional Paraguayan foods as healthful and desirable, some also worried that these calorie-dense foods were ill-suited to the modern economy. As fifty-one-year-old night watchman Jorge explained, "Our culture, it's all heavy foods. From childhood our parents fed us like this, and now we too carry this culture … it would be good to change this lifestyle." Others disagreed, arguing that the problem was that people were no longer consuming traditional foods. Elisa, the forty-nine-year-old wife of Juan the tailor, said, "People on low incomes eat them, but wealthy people don't eat *puchero* (stew with bone/marrow), they don't eat *vorí*." And as Jorge's fifty-two-year-old wife, Antonia, saw it, "We eat badly … Look, every few steps you see junk food. Everywhere, and now people don't want to cook anymore … They take out a pizza or a hamburger or order this and that. Generally, it's for convenience."

The reasons given for the popularity of fast food varied, but people often pointed to economic and social structural problems. Some said that the frenetic pace of modern life leaves little time to shop and cook healthy foods. Sergei, a forty-four-year-old mechanic explained,

> It is easier for parents to go buy precooked food, some *milanesa* (breaded fried meat) you can just give your family, something fast … To me, this is just fast food, junk food. Yes, because it is easier to go to the supermarket, buy precooked food by the kilo, and put it on the table for your child.

Others said that healthy foods are more expensive than fast foods. Jorge said: "Here it's really expensive if you want to eat healthy. Fruits, vegetables, all that – it comes out much more expensive to feed a family." Maima, a twenty-year-old stay-at-home mother with two children, explained that buying healthy restaurant food is not a financial feasibility for most families: "There are very few places that sell healthy food. Yeah, luxury restaurants, but they are too expensive. *Empanadas* (savory turnovers), hamburgers, and that stuff: those are the least expensive restaurants you are going to find in Encarnación." In these ways, the high cost of quality foods, the time required to cook, and the lack of healthy alternatives all contributed to creating an obesogenic environment in Encarnación.

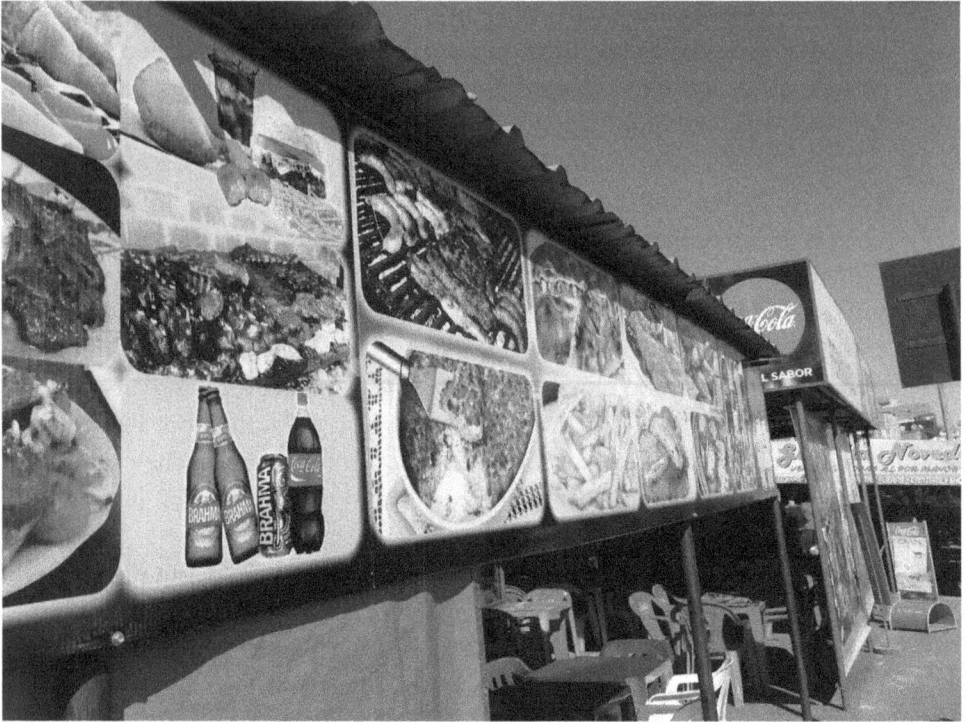

Figure 5.2. A typical fast food restaurant in the market, with signs advertising *asado* (BBQ), *empanadas* (savory turnovers), *sopa paraguaya* (cornbread), hamburgers, fries, soda, and beer

At a broader level, recent patterns in migration, displacement, and resettlement have also reshaped many families' foodways. In the last decade, many rural Paraguayan smallholders have been driven off their land by big soy plantation owners. Forced to come to the city, often penniless, many rural migrants rely on a diet of cheap fast foods. Sofia, a wealthy and well-educated fifty-eight-year-old woman descended from Paraguayan political dissidents, told Amber:

> Before people ate well. But now that's been left behind. Because big business is so powerful here that they took the poor people's land and forced the poor into the city, creating an enormous poverty zone. You see how it is, people come from the countryside where before they had cows, pigs, chickens, eggs, cheese, everything. They came here with nothing

when the big agribusinesses took their land. Then everything
changed. Now they eat garbage and the transnationals gorge
themselves on money. That's how it is.

Similarly, people displaced by the Yacyretá Dam lost access to land
they used for growing gardens and raising small farm animals. Without these sources of home-grown healthy foods, they say, they eat less
healthily than they once did.

Many people completely dismissed structural reasons for being
fat. They said the overconsumption of fast foods was just a problem
born of sheer laziness. As Antonia (the fifty-two-year-old housewife
and part-time cleaning woman) said: "Young people don't want to
cook anymore. Look, they'd rather go take out a pizza than have to
buy and make white rice and have to sauté meat." This idea – the one
that faults people's laziness for dietary changes – was one of the most
common explanations for rising obesity rates in Paraguay. Between
1975 and 2013, the obesity rate in Paraguay has increased from around
5 per cent to over 20 per cent of the adult population.[8] As of 2016,
46 per cent of Paraguay's population was overweight and 15 per cent
was Obese.[9] A good proportion of these are children; in 2011, an esti-
mated 20 per cent of Paraguayan children were Obese.[10] Paraguayans
are, of course, well aware of this demographic shift and many are worried about it. When asked who is responsible for Paraguayans' weight
gain, nearly everyone says weight gain is a personal responsibility.

Paraguayans tend to see weight loss as a personal responsibility, too.
When talking about others, they explain that each person is responsible for their own eating choices. As Estefanía, a twenty-nine-year-old
woman who ran a fast food restaurant, said, "I think it depends on
each person ... Even though there are lots of fast food restaurants here,
there are also many places where someone can eat something healthier. I think it depends on each person, and that's just how it is." Similarly, people often said that motivation to exercise and lose weight
must come from within. Pacha, a thirty-three-year-old businessman,
said, "The family can help, but if the overweight or underweight person does not take care of himself, nobody can do anything for him ...
So, in my view, that same person has to be the one to give himself
the encouragement to lose weight or to feel good about himself." The
idea that people were personally responsible for their weight was

expressed in many ways, but it was a common one expressed across the interviews conducted in Encarnación.

Yet when Amber asked about family members or friends – loved ones who seemed to struggle with their weight – people were noticeably less likely to point the finger in blame. Reflective of the strong commitment to social support that is common in Paraguay,[11] many said that they felt responsible for ensuring that family and friends had the support they needed to lose weight. Juan – the forty-nine-year-old tailor – said, "In our community, we need to care for each other, right? We have to tell each other, 'Fulana [so-and-so], you need to lose some more weight.' Or, 'Fulano, you need to lose weight for your health.' To give each other advice."

Amber often interviewed people who discussed ways they could help their loved ones: by exercising together with a friend, changing their own diet to help a family member make healthy food choices, or simply being supportive of them. Some respondents noted that overeating was a common symptom of stress and depression and explained the need to help others overcome mental distress. In marriages, these patterns of mutual social support around weight, exercise, and wellness were especially visible. Juan (the tailor) and Elisa talked about making time to exercise together. Neider (the clothes vendor) and Sergei explained how they plan each week's healthy meals and grocery shop together. Jorge (the night watchman) and Antonia economized together so that they could both afford to go to the nutritionist. Thus, while weight judgments and personal blame were common in Encarnación, they were balanced by people's commitment to support their loved ones in adopting better diets, exercising more frequently, and, it is hoped, maintaining a healthy weight.

WHEN IS FAT BAD? "YOU'VE GOT HYPERTENSION, DIABETES, CIRCULATORY ILLNESSES ..."

Encarnacenos tend to believe that they do not discriminate based on weight. Again and again, Amber heard respondents insist that being overweight would not harm anyone's life chances. As Neider, the thirty-seven-year-old clothes vendor, said, "No. Discrimination because someone is fat? We see very little of that here ... it's good because there is no discrimination for anyone. It could be for fat people; or it could be because they are dark-skinned or *negrito* [Black], as they say ... You see, people in Encarnación don't discriminate much." Being a bit overweight, most people explained, would not affect someone's ability to find a mate. Most people also said that being overweight almost never affected someone's ability to get a job. As Pacha, a thirty-three-year-old businessman, said, "Here it's not like in other countries where they have a strong concept of discrimination. Most people take it as a joke." Denise, a thirty-five-year-old cardiologist's assistant, said: "What's happening is that we Paraguayans ... we're a relaxed people. We don't complain; we don't say anything; we accept. That's it, we're relaxed, because nobody is going to say 'Ay! This is discrimination.' I might make a comment to you as my friend ... but it stays between us, and nothing ever changes."

The one exception was in service industry employment – for example, a front-desk attendant, bank teller, high-end sales-clerk, and other public-facing office jobs. For such jobs, there was a general agreement that having a *buena presencia* (literally "good presence," meaning thin, good-looking, well-dressed) was a prerequisite to employment. When Amber asked Sofia, the thin, wealthy fifty-eight-year-old woman whose adult children were all high-status professionals, about this, she swiftly seized that day's newspaper and rifled through the "help wanted" ads. Finding one that called for buena presencia, Sofia pointed it out and said, "People who have good jobs in certain places, like banks, in finance, they have to worry about having good bodies, nice clothes, being well-groomed ... If you go to a bank, or for financial services, or an insurance company, you are not going to see ugly girls or fat girls. No, these people do a ton to maintain their bodies." Interestingly, Pacha, a wealthy and successful businessman, said almost the same thing as Sofia, word for word.

Yet, Maima, the twenty-year-old stay-at-home mother who called herself overweight, disagreed about the extremity of these body norms: "*Buena presencia* matters. It's not just in the bank. To work anywhere here, they ask you for *buena presencia* now. I mean, I do not say skinny or anything, but, well-dressed, well-groomed, nice teeth. I'm not saying perfect, but a little cute. Yes, *buena presencia*. Well-groomed and all that." Others, with larger bodies or less class status, agreed more with Maima than the upper-class participants, Sofia and Pacha.

Amber observed that people's class status and body weight seemed to shape how they interpreted the meaning and severity of these body norms for employment, but there was no question that buena presencia mattered for getting and keeping some jobs.

Yet despite these hints of thin-idealism and possible employment discrimination, some respondents argued that being a bit rounded out *could* be considered attractive. To probe a bit more at this tricky point, Amber asked women about their experiences with men who engage in what Paraguayans call a *piropo*.[12] Piropos often take the form of a poetic ode to a woman's beauty, sometimes raunchy, sometimes comically flowery, shouted at a woman walking down the street. Large-bodied women, Amber was told, can receive piropos that are very complimentary. For example, thirty-five-year-old Mia recounted fondly the piropos of her adolescence:

> Out walking with my sister, men would always say, "Ay, I like the plump one!" right? It was pleasant. One time my sister got mad: "Geez, fatty," she said, "you always get the *piropos* – and what about me?" She'd say this to me because I was chubby. But I was always likable, happy. In contrast, my sister was thin, but she had a face that was very serious, mean, apathetic. So, they'd always appreciate my amiability, my – what do I know? – my smile. It was more than my physical appearance. And anyway, I wasn't very fat. I was plump, filled-in.

Yet, Paraguayans love double meanings and piropos containing the word *gorda* are a perfect example of this. Gorda (and its dimunitive *gordita*) can be translated as fat, fatty, overweight, plump, chubby, filled-in. As Ferdinando, a thirty-five-year-old retired professional soccer player – who agreed, based on his longtime friendship with Amber, to tell her the awkward and embarrassing truths nobody else wanted to explain – said, "We Paraguayans can be quite nasty sometimes … capable of saying, 'Here comes the fatty.' Gordo or gorda (fat) is a word that can be used as much for affection as it is for that [to offend]." In this way, gorda (and gordita) can be used simultaneously as a compliment and an insult. Piropos are not unambiguously complimentary: veiled as compliments, they can be used to call attention to women's large bodies and humiliate them. As this example of piropos shows, there is a deep ambivalence around large bodies – especially large-bodied women – lurking just underneath the surface insistence of body acceptance and non-discrimination in Paraguay.

Paraguayans will freely admit to mocking and joking with people about their bodies. In Encarnación, it was often said that people are quite blunt about telling someone they are overweight. Fat jokes are also very common. For example, Neider, the thirty-seven-year-old clothes vendor explained, "You'd go to the pool and it was like you had to be skinny, or else people would stare at you and laugh." Not everyone agreed that such jokes were amusing. As Pacha, the thirty-three-year-old businessman said, "So, imagine somebody is fat. Because they are fat, people won't call them by their name. They just call them 'Gordo' ... In Paraguay, we are not very advanced in our understanding of 'bullying,' as they say." It's worth noting that Pacha said the word "bullying" in English – further emphasizing that this is a foreign concept, recently imported into Paraguayan parlance. While Neider and Pacha make a strong case that fat jokes are hurtful, most people characterized fat jokes about adults (but not children) as good fun, and further evidence that Paraguayans were not overly sensitive about weight. Interestingly, people often said that they switch into Guaraní when they wanted to make a fat joke, especially to someone's face. Pacha explained, "Whenever someone makes a mean joke, they say *gordo* [in Guaraní]." Sergei the mechanic, too, affirmed that these joking commentaries would be "in Guaraní. They say, for example, [in Guaraní] that fatty can't even move." When Amber asked why people preferred to switch to Guaraní to make such commentaries, nearly everyone agreed it was because Guaraní is "harsher" than Spanish.

Paraguayans' use of social media can intensify this cruelty, several people told Amber. "Recently, on social media, the 'blue whale' was making the rounds," said Mia, the thirty-five-year-old woman who recalled the piropos of her youth. "For example, everybody's at a party and they say 'Hey, here comes the blue whale!' They say it to you as you are arriving, for example – they compare you with a whale, right? Supposedly it's a joke – to make people laugh at others, right?" Then, Mia gets to the heart of the issue: "Here, jokes are used a lot" for fat shaming, Mia explained. "The insults come in the form of jokes all the time. But people are really saying what they want to say – but in the form of a joke." While these jokes and insults show ways in which fat people are devalued, there is more at play. Paraguayans also see increasing obesity rates as ominous visible evidence of the negative impacts of unwanted cultural and economic changes. In these ways, Paraguayans see obese people as embodying all the things they fear becoming: forced into a fast-paced economy, lacking free-time, neglecting family and community, and turning their backs on culture and tradition.

Perhaps unsurprisingly, when Amber questioned them a bit more deeply, people did admit that perhaps encarnacenos with large bodies did feel badly about themselves. Respondents generally characterized this as self-stigma – feelings of shame and failure that people impose on themselves – rather than stigma forced onto them by the negative judgments and treatment of others. Juan, in his work as a tailor, had often observed people's embarrassment at their size when measuring them for alterations and new clothes. Juan explained:

> With men it's not much, and they don't care. They come, I take their measurements, and they don't complain much. Because they tell you, "I need to lose more weight." And they never do, and that's it. And we always joke about it, yes, yes, yes. A woman is different. The women see things differently ... some of them complain that they are *gordita* [fat]. When it's a young lady, then she'll really complain a bit and have a bit of embarrassment. But I always tell them, "Don't be ashamed," and I try to find a way to ensure they don't feel badly about themselves.

Such feelings, people told Amber, caused some women to withdraw socially. People generally characterized the choice to stay home from celebrations and parties as an expression of shame and discomfort. But people also recognized that obesity, shame, and stigma can be closely linked to poor mental health. As Zulma, a slim forty-seven-year-old woman who ran her own small business, said, "People have unhealthy lives ... It's the reality. And they are lazy ... many people get depressed because of this ... I have many girlfriends, acquaintances, cousins – they get depressed." Further, several people recognized that overeating can be linked to stress or a symptom of depression. People seemed to understand that obesity and mental illness could be linked in a cyclical pattern: people overeat because they are stressed; they become socially isolated because they are overweight; social isolation can create depression. In these ways, obesity was seen by some respondents as potentially linked to poor mental health.

More broadly recognized were the links between obesity and poor physical health. Many respondents said that they had recently adopted new diet and exercise routines because they wanted to get healthy. Others said they feared that they would develop high blood pressure or diabetes or feared for family members who had done so. People's fears about the health impacts of obesity are intensified by the tough realities of obesity treatment in Paraguay. Paraguay, like most countries around the world (rich or poor), has a nationalized health-care system. In Encarnación, health care is delivered through the IPS, or Instituto de Previsión Social (Social Security Institute), for people with formal employment. While the IPS is a public health-care system, access to care was notoriously inaccessible. Jorge (the fifty-one-year-old night watchman) said, that when you get sick, "you have to go at 3:00, 3:30 in the morning to wait, and there's already a huge line. Sometimes you get to the front of the line, ask to speak to a professional, and they say, 'No, there are no more spots today.'" Elisa, Juan the tailor's forty-nine-year-old wife, explained how she navigates the medical system in Encarnación: "I don't go to IPS [hospitals]. I have my [IPS] insurance, but I also have another insurance that I pay for privately ... IPS is very chaotic. My daughter went once when she was sick, and nobody paid any attention to her; she had to leave and come back." In Paraguay, wealthy and upper-middle-class families enjoy high-quality private providers and insurance plans. Yet informally employed Paraguayans (like street vendors or part-time maids and caregivers) do not even have access to IPS – often, they must pay for care out of pocket.

For people seeking to lose weight or suffering obesity-related health conditions, obtaining medical treatment was a great burden. Denise, a thirty-five-year-old woman who worked in a cardiac clinic, described her patients' health problems: "You've got hypertension, diabetes, circulatory illnesses, for example, cholesterol, triglycerides, and joint pain." All of these require costly monitoring and medicine. Pacha, the wealthy thirty-three-year-old businessman, said that obesity coverage was only available to people with expensive private insurance. "You can get your trainer and your nutritionist paid for – by private insurance. Most [upper-]middle-class people have private medical insurance," Pacha explained. Given the lack of publicly funded support for obesity treatments, Amber wondered what less well-off people were doing for weight-loss support. When she asked, the most common response was "go to a nutritionist."

Nutritionist services in Encarnación typically include regular advice consultations, the creation and monitoring of a personalized diet and weight plan, the purchase of a specialized diet (which often includes home delivery), and sometimes the prescribing of diet medications. Since health foods and diet foods are rarely sold in Paraguayan supermarkets, nutritionists are one of the few sources of low-calorie and low-fat foods. Even respondents who were only slightly overweight explained that they were under the care of a nutritionist – when they could afford it.

As Denise, the thirty-five-year-old cardiologist's assistant, said: "I have my lunches delivered. For the last two months I've been eating healthy, not much beef or fried food, right? I wanted to start to lose some weight ... I am about 6 kilos [13 pounds] overweight." Neider, the thirty-seven-year-old clothes vendor, described what it's like to diet in Encarnación:

> Dieting here is, let's say, not cheap. No – a diet meal would cost something like 15,000 guaraníes [US$2.50] for a plate of food ... Yes, really healthy food, like a nutritionist would make – between meals, dinner, and everything – more or less comes to 100,000 guaraníes [US$16] a day ... there are many nutritionists here in Encarnación. But some give you a diet that you follow, but there are others that do the cooking themselves. Then they send you the food.

These specialized foods, sold and delivered by nutritionists, can be quite expensive, especially for lower-middle-class and impoverished families. Antonia, a fifty-two-year-old housewife and part-time cleaning woman Amber met through a private nutritionist, explained:

> I don't do what my nutritionist tells me, because if I'm going to do as he tells me ... what my nutritionist says is too expensive. It costs a lot of money to follow a diet, because he orders you a chicken, a salad, everything is dietetic and diet foods are

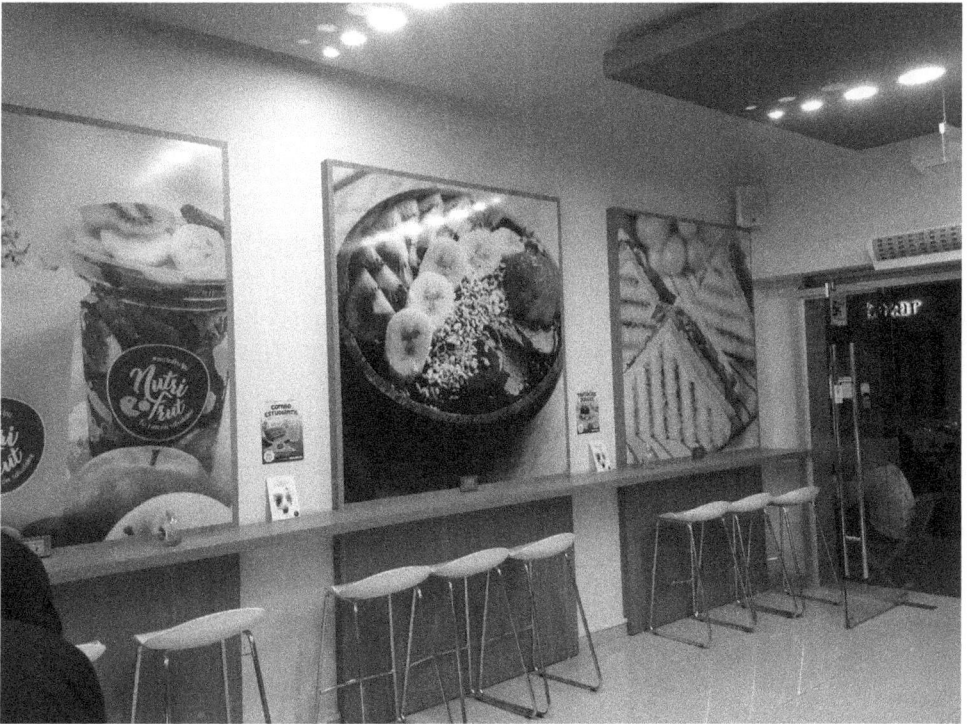

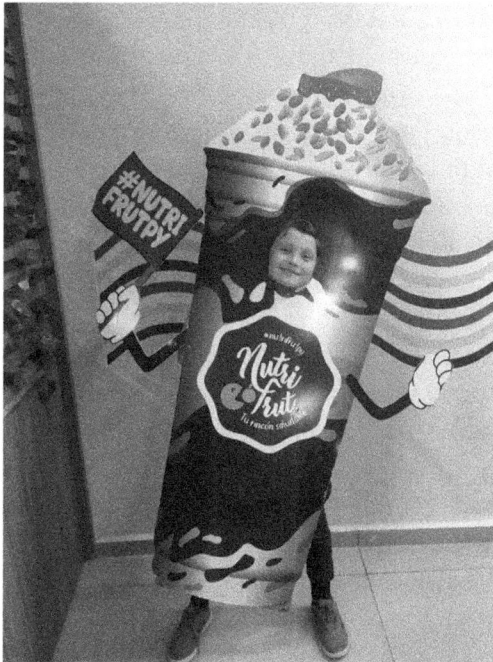

Figure 5.3. In a trendy new health food restaurant in Encarnación (top), Amber's son Alexandro tries on a promotional sign (bottom)

> expensive. But they know and they try to accommodate you.
> Well, for example, he says, "Well, if you cannot buy this, then
> switch it and eat this."

The nutritionist explained that many people felt they had to make the financial sacrifice of paying for nutritional counseling and services, given the serious health risks and long-term costs associated with diabetes, heart disease, and other obesity-related health conditions. Further, the cost of weight-loss treatments and obesity-related health care meant many overweight middle-class and lower-middle-class Paraguayans were forced to navigate a complex patchwork of public and private health services. Jorge the night watchman, who is also Antonia's husband, explained:

> For us, going to a private doctor isn't impossible, but it's really
> expensive, right? You think, if I pay for this now, later I won't
> have money for things my kid needs, and all those kinds of
> concerns. So mostly we have to rely on public health care, but
> our situation there is very precarious. It's practically ... how
> can I say this? ... it doesn't meet our expectations. The quality
> of care – it's not that. Rather, the issue is, for example, med-
> ications: There's never enough of anything. They don't have
> them. So you have to buy them [out of pocket], and often
> you're not in a financial position to buy them. Because, I tell
> you, there's not enough money, just not enough. So we go
> without medications. And really, the quality of care is really ...
> I don't know how to explain it ... the professionals are unpro-
> fessional. Really. They don't get it. Maybe it's just that they've
> never had to experience anything like this themselves, right?
> But here in Paraguay there are a lot of people who aren't fi-
> nancially able to go to a private clinic or doctor.

As Jorge's comments show, most people Amber talked to felt that the public health-care system was to be used as a last resort for the treatment of obesity-related conditions like high blood pressure or diabetes. All agreed that there was essentially no treatment available for obesity prevention in the public health-care system. In most cases, people had to scrimp and save to be able to pay for high-quality obesity prevention and treatment from private doctors and nutritionists.

And, of course, those who did not qualify for IPS and other forms of public coverage, often the most impoverished, had to pay for all obesity-related treatments totally out of pocket. This meant that they only got care when their need was truly severe.

Paraguay, like many countries with high rates of inequality, has a dual burden of obesity and food insecurity. Some respondents explained that, unlike obesity care, public assistance was available to address food insecurity. As Luján, a wealthy twenty-eight-year-old businesswoman married to Pacha, explained, "The focus is more on malnutrition, because there is a lot of malnutrition here. In the lower classes, for example, malnutrition is common. But there's nothing like this for obese people. In Argentina, for example, they have treatment plans for people who are obese, for obesity, all of that. I've never heard of that happening here." Maima, the twenty-year-old mother of two, was the only person Amber interviewed who received supplemental food services. She said: "I have IPS insurance, through my husband, and you can go there for free and they have many, many nutritionists … my [three-month-old] daughter drank [infant formula] milk thanks to the nutritionists … they give you milk, and every month we'd go with my daughter and they'd weigh her, and check her to see that she was doing well." In Paraguay, respondents unhappily explained, malnutrition is considered a legitimate part of the public health system, while obesity is a privatized health risk.

While sharp critiques of Paraguay's public health system were common, only a few respondents suggested broader structural solutions to the obesity problem. When Amber asked about different kinds of possible regulatory measures, such as taxing unhealthy foods or creating exercise opportunities at a community level, very little enthusiasm was expressed. For example, when Amber asked Juan, the forty-nine-year-old tailor, "Could the community play a role in addressing obesity?" he replied: "Here, no. No, no, no. No." This negative response was fairly common, reflecting a general sense that addressing obesogenic environments was beyond the scope and capability of the government. One exception was Luján, who felt that the government "could do more to enforce regulations … there's very little oversight of pubs and hamburger joints. They're on every half block, and they are so convenient and cheap. If the government did more to enforce good regulations, they wouldn't be so common." Yet people more frequently had the attitude that the government would be useless in confronting obesity, and that it could only be addressed through medical and individual efforts. For example, Rosa, a sixty-year-old retired principal, said, "I have diabetes. I'm overweight. I'm not taking care of myself … I'm not doing what's right, and I know I'm not. I need to lower my sugar levels." Most people who told Amber they were overweight or had obesity-related illnesses shared Rosa's conviction that their extra weight was their own fault, and that it was their responsibility to change and improve their health. Rosa's nutritionist, too, told Amber that most encarnacenos just needed to make more of an effort to improve their health education, change their diets, and increase their exercise. Such views were widely shared among people in Encarnación.

WHO IS FAT? "PARAGUAYAN BODIES ARE 'NORMAL'"

Historically, nearly everyone agreed, thinness in Paraguay was common and a sign of poverty and hunger. Mia said,

> In those times, there was less obesity … Paraguay was very poor. Food scarcity, I think, had a role because in the times of my uncles and aunts – people I've known and whose youth I have seen in photos – people were thin. My grandmother, for example, was thin until after she had her fourth child, more or less. They lived in extreme poverty in the countryside, and later they moved to the city and my grandfather and grandmother were both able to work. Then, they began to have more economic stability, and my grandmother's body grew larger.

As with Mia's family, many people acknowledged that, as Paraguay became more economically stable, people migrated to urban centers, food security improved, wealth accumulated, and bodies grew larger.

What is a Paraguayan body like today? If you ask people in Encarnación, they'll tell you Paraguayan bodies are "normal" – neither too fat, nor too thin. Extreme obesity and thinness are relatively rare, according to regular residents and clinicians. The nutritionist Amber interviewed said, for example, that very few of his clients are "morbidly obese" with over 100 kilos (220 pounds) or even 50 kilos (110 pounds) of excess weight. Rather, he said that most were just overweight.

While body norms were characterized as somewhat loose for every-one, there was general agreement that men had it easier. Yet there was also wide acknowledgment that body norms were changing for men. While a bit of a beer belly is still considered permissible, well-cut muscular bodies are considered increasingly desirable. As Denise, the thirty-five-year-old cardiologist's assistant, said, "Here, for men, it's not so ... not so ... how do you say? ... not so meticulous. It's more relaxed with men. A little. Not so much." Mia, a mother of teenage sons, explained knowledgeably, "There are a lot of overweight men ... people make fun of them ... So now the ones who want to be thin, skinny, muscular, they go to the gym. Because the girls these days are really demanding – in my day, it wasn't really like that."

Even as men's bodies come under greater scrutiny, everyone agreed that body ideals and beauty norms were more stringent for women. Ferdinando, the retired soccer player, described Paraguayan women's ideal body as rounded-out with "good breasts, a nice bootie, and a good waist." The nutritionist concurred, saying that 80 per cent of his cli-entele are women who come for aesthetic reasons. There is definitely more pressure for encarnacena women to conform to more interna-tional beauty norms, the nutritionist continued, because Encarnación is one of Paraguay's more sophisticated and wealthy cities. Encarnacenos are very much oriented to the beauty standards of Argentina, which sits just across the Paraná River. So, to conform to those standards, the nutritionist said, the women among his clientele want and need to diet.

Not everyone agrees that Paraguayans should adopt the extreme Argentine beauty standards indiscriminately. In fact, there is quite a bit of pushback against them among encarnacenos. As Mia – the for-mer owner of a plus-size clothing business – explains, Paraguayan body ideals are:

> To be slender: neither too thin, nor too fat. These ideas come from outside of Paraguay. Here in Encarnación, it's Argentine culture ... in Cuidad del Este, it's Brazilian influence. In gen-eral, in these countries, the stereotype for women is a thin body. Slender, tall – generally. The Paraguayan woman is very balanced. She has, generally, a nice bust and a nice bottom. In comparison, Argentine women have a nice bust but no bot-tom, and Brazilian women have a bottom but no bust. The

> Paraguayan woman is generally at an intermediate point be-
> tween these two. I spent many years selling clothes, so I know
> the figure of Argentine women and the fit of their clothes.

Cosmetic surgery is increasingly talked about in Encarnación. Luján, the wealthy twenty-eight-year-old businesswoman, said, "Most people do their breasts or their noses; I have two friends who have. I did it too … In Brazil, I did *lipo* [liposuction] and *dermo* [skin removal] after having my baby … I had a lot of leftover fat, and I fell into something of a depression." While cosmetic surgery had become common in Luján's social circle, it was unimaginable for many middle-class and lower-middle-class people Amber interviewed. When Amber asked Denise, the cardiologist's assistant, if she'd want to change her body, she gave a more typical reply: "Yes, I think I should lose more weight. But with respect to operations, some kind of surgery? No." Similarly, people see extreme obesity, and bariatric surgery, as foreign imports. In sharp contrast to what encarnacenos characterize as their own body-accepting and community-oriented ways, they characterize their nearest foreign neighbors – Argentines and Brazilians – as extreme-bodied, body-obsessed, and the importers of foreign body ideals. Nevertheless, these "foreign practices" are slowly making their way into Encarnación, especially for younger people.

While young encarnacenos feel some pressure to adhere to ideal body norms, Paraguayan bodies are understood to naturally change substantially over the lifespan. Participants offered different sayings to capture this truism. Neider, the thirty-seven-year-old mother who sells clothes in the market, said, "Much changes, as in the famous saying, '*Te casaste y engordaste*' [You got married and you got fat]." Ferdinado quoted a cruder saying that captures even more vividly this expected and accepted transformation: "*90, 60, 90 que te revienta.*" The numbers 90–60–90 refer to the ideal measurements for women in centimeters (much like the so-called 36–24–36 inch ideal), and *que te revienta* means, more or less, "will burst on you." Like so many beloved jokes in Paraguay, this one has a double meaning. The first meaning is that a woman with ideal measurements will make a man *reventar* (ejaculate). The second meaning is that the woman with ideal measurements will *reventar* (blow up by getting really fat). The joke is that the woman becomes less sexually desirable as she ages, but the general attitude – much like the sentiment expressed by Samira at the start of this chapter – is that this is expected and is no big deal.

If adult obesity is no big deal, the opposite is true of child obesity: it is a very big deal to encarnaceno parents. Most frightening are people's worries for their own children and relatives, many of whom were already showing signs of childhood obesity. Maima, the twenty-year-old stay-at-home mom, said, for example:

> I have a cousin who is eight years old and weighs like 60 kilos [132 pounds]; he's overweight and really fat. And nobody says anything to him, because like all parents – it pains you if somebody comes and tells you your son is fat. His mom takes him to a nutritionist to try to manage it. But he is really – he has a lot of anxiety.

Pacha, who worries about his two-year-old child's weight, said,

> These days things are much tougher ... Don't play with the *gordo*, don't talk to the *gordo*, don't lend your homework to the *gordo*. But this – before, it wasn't like this. I mean, we teased the *gordo*, but we never made him feel left out. We never did this – we never excluded him ... It's getting worse, yes.

Mia, who struggled with her own weight over the years, said:

> My son – the biggest one – who is about to turn fifteen. As a child, he was a bit obese. And always I tried to watch his diet, to help him, to teach him, right? ... For his health above all, and for the discrimination that there is against obese people. Because I experienced it and I know in school the children are very cruel.

Some parents were worried not just about their children's experiences in school but also about their future life chances. Sergei, the forty-four-year-old mechanic and husband of Neider, said: "My [nine-year-old] daughter – I see she's affected when people tell her she's fat, like in her dance troupe, right? It affects her a bit." Sergei went on to worry that obesity could affect his daughter's future: "She's intelligent and all that, and if she doesn't have the ideal body for a certain job, I think that would upset her for sure." Even respondents who did not have an overweight child at home voiced strong fears for the future health of obese Paraguayan children.

INTERVIEWING AND EATING IN ENCARNACIÓN

Food and fat were interwoven through the interactions Amber had with people in Encarnación. Amber felt fortunate to have been invited to share meals with many of the people in the study. Eating together – in homes, restaurants, and cafés – provided a space for Amber to explore what food meant to people's lives and their bodies. Participant-observation enriched Amber's understandings of the meanings of food and fat.

The many meals shared with study participants provided Amber with crucial insights. For example, Amber came to understand that food refusal was a socially powerful form of rejection for people in Encarnación. Amber's first inkling of this was when she was told a favorite story – one that had clearly been humorously told and retold – about a terrible relative who refused the off-brand soda when it was offered. Amber, who is not a big soda drinker, scrambled to apologize for past soda refusals. She was reassured: it wasn't that the terrible relative wouldn't drink soda, but that she said *only name-brand soda* would do *to our faces*! After this, Amber was highly attuned to food refusals and their meanings. A refusal to share Samira's meal after her godson's baptism signaled that someone did not want to be considered part of the family. A refusal to accept food that was prepared for a family member who was sick was a hurtful rejection. A refusal to eat street food prepared by two street vendors was an assertion of class status. Most of these events came to Amber through jokes and humorous storytelling – a powerful demonstration of how meaning is made and socially reinforced in Encarnación.

Yet these insights could never have emerged without a foundation of strong and trusting relationships, into which the data collection and interpretation was woven. When Amber interviewed Sofia, for example, Sofia prepared an impromptu lunch of ham omelets and salad for Amber's children and spouse. This moment of care was one of Amber's many cherished memories from that summer in Encarnación. Such experiences highlight the importance of deep and long-standing community engagements for research on sensitive topics like food and fat.

CHAPTER SIX

Lapo'a (Large) in Apia, Samoa

The café is noisy. The coffee machine cranks as beans are freshly ground for flat whites and long blacks. The machine grinds and clicks so loudly that Jessica worries her recording won't be audible. The blender buzzes making papaya, banana, and basil smoothies. Kilisi (age forty-two) and her husband, Loto (age forty-eight), arrive, squeezing into a corner table, and explain that they only have about three days on-island before they have to leave again. Kilisi works for a United States agency; fears of "slashed budgets" means she had to fly to Washington, DC, for a three-week training session. Her boss had notified her only a few days earlier. She had just returned from New Zealand days before where she was visiting her brother, who was struggling with alcoholism, complicated by his diabetes. His alcohol use, and his diabetes diagnosis, started when their father died six years ago. Kilisi flew to New Zealand to relieve her other siblings and make sure her nieces and nephews were cared for. They weren't. Despite all this, Kilisi embraced Jessica with a long tight hug, as they hadn't seen each other since about five years previously.

The café Jessica suggested was "upmarket," owned by a well-known culinary family who operated other successful restaurants nearby. The glass glimmered, the tables were filled with well-known faces, and the staff greeted everyone warmly, offering a newspaper to some or a box of toys to nannies who accompanied families. When Jessica asked potential interviewees where they would prefer to meet, they would defer to her. Then, when Jessica mentioned she was paying for lunch, they sometimes shyly suggested this café. Jessica ordered an omelet, Loto ordered *oka* and poke – both raw fish dishes – and Kilisi ordered a spinach and feta omelet. Later she'd joke that she didn't like vegetables. Jessica ribbed, "But you ordered the veggie omelet?!" Kilisi laughed, "I wanted to impress you."

Over lunch, Kilisi reflected on how meals had changed since she was a girl. She remembered having just two meals a day growing up. Boiled green bananas bathed in coconut cream, usually left from the night before, served as "breakfast" after morning chores were complete. These bananas became the base for a late evening meal. They were both big meals, made from a few ingredients – starches, coconut cream, sometimes meat. Everything came from their garden – the chickens, the banana, and the coconuts used for *koko risa* (rice cooked with local varieties of cacao). Now, Kilisi preferred to eat takeout in the evenings, like chicken stir fry with *sopisui*, the Samoan term for chop suey. Loto, however, insisted on health first, and wanted home-cooked meals rich with vegetables. But Kilisi managed the household budget meticulously, insisting that buying takeout was cheaper than getting enough vegetables, which they had to buy, to feed the whole house to satiety.

Loto described his childhood meals by saying, that in their own garden, "We had almost everything." This diet was the key to Samoan health, he said. He reflected that even though their bodies were large, his family worked hard, so their size was "normal," he was careful to say. He reminded Jessica, Polynesians typically have larger bodies than *palagi* (white) people, but they were healthy because they stayed fit with chores like chopping firewood, planting and harvesting crops, shaving coconuts to make cream, and digging an *umu* (earth oven). Now, with so many people working in offices, like Kilisi, there was no time to do this work or land to grow food. Health suffered.

The other most popular location for interviews was in the lobby of Aggie Grey's Sheraton Hotel (see figure 6.1). A staple in Apia since the 1930s, famed and recently renovated, the air-conditioned lobby was comfortable, in a corporate way. The furniture was heavy, featuring beige cushions on dark wood, and each time Jessica walked through the revolving doors, she wondered how all that stuff got there. She'd imagine shipping containers filled with generic hotel furniture and large lobby rugs. Before the recent renovation, the lobby was open-air

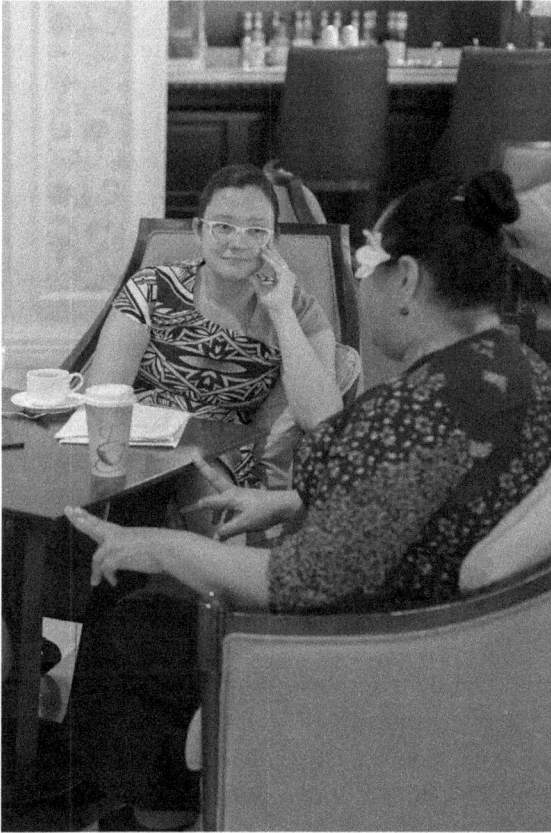

Figure 6.1. Jessica interviewing one of the women in the lobby of Aggie Grey's Sheraton Hotel

and decorated with hand-painted gold coconuts, now replaced with heavy bar stools, stone counters, and glass cabinets filled with expensive imported liquors – Kahlúa, Jameson, Smirnoff. Women Jessica didn't know very well often recommended meeting in the lobby, saying it was air-conditioned (and therefore probably comfortable for Jessica, as a palagi foreigner). Always on her second or third coffee of the day, Jessica would switch to tea and would often be served a pot, English style in white porcelain. Jessica's company would order tea or coffee, and then she'd splurge on brownies or banana bread to make the meeting feel sweeter.

These places, urban corporate hotels and high-end cafés frequented by Samoans and not tourists, might not reflect what you imagine when you think about Polynesia. These places, in fact, were vital to everyday life among cosmopolitan Samoans. Yet they are often invisible in large-scale epidemiological studies that explain dietary change in terms of increased calorie consumption and decreased physical activity.

Of the twenty-four people Jessica interviewed for this study, ten were couples (she interviewed five sets of husbands and wives). In total, she interviewed five men and nineteen women: eight of the nineteen women were married and eleven were not married. All but one interviewee lived with extended family that included parents, grandparents, aunts, uncles, and children. Family was at the center of many of the stories people told. This chapter highlights the social life of foods and fat to show that fat isn't clearly bad or good; instead, context matters in shaping how ordinary people evaluate the relationship between weight, eating, and feeding.

PERI-URBAN SAMOA: SOME CONTEXT

Samoa is an independent nation. But it is also culturally part of a larger island group that includes the US territory of American Samoa. The capital city of Apia is on the largest island in the archipelago; the city unfolds around Beach Road, lined with monuments, markets, hotels, and government buildings. In the past decade, there has been steady growth, as measured by the sheer number of new buildings. Shopping plazas, gyms, government offices, and cafés have multiplied in recent years. This has been matched by growth in the health sector, including a new hospital, public health offices, and a medical school. When Jessica asked people about the sudden popularity of cafés, they would scoff, it's returning migrants, bringing their money and urban culture from New Zealand. The upmarket cafés, with expensive imported espresso machines were matched by brand-new pickup trucks growling up hills to family compounds, guarded by fences and fat, sleek dogs. But Apia also has stark contrasts, with modest wood houses without walls tucked away behind main roads, also guarded by dogs, though these tend to be hungrier and mangier.

Over 20 per cent of Samoa's 200,000 population lives in Apia, a very recent shift from an almost entirely rural lifestyle.[1] However, urban life is no less shaped by *fa'a samoa* (Samoan culture, the

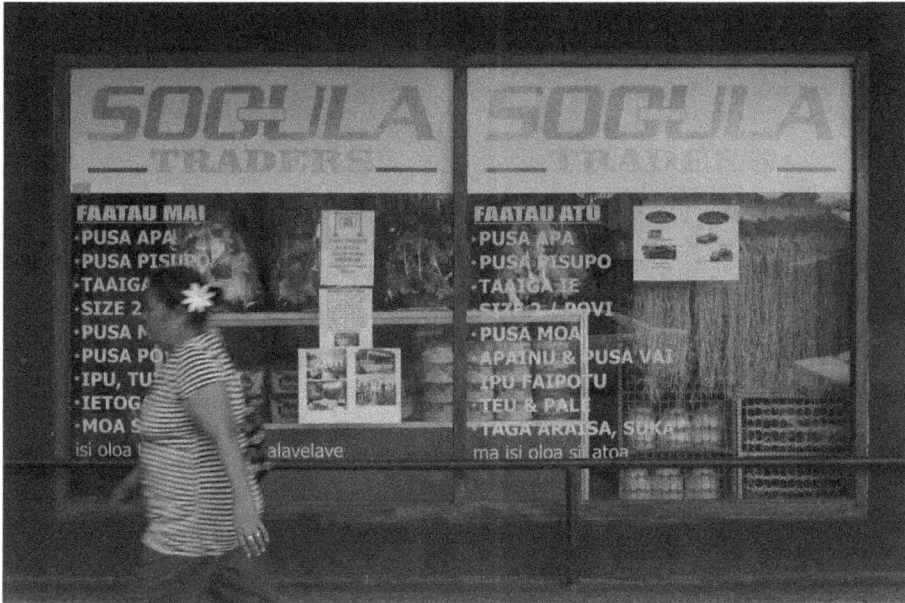

Figure 6.2. A shop dedicated to items required for *fa'alavelave*

Samoan way) than elsewhere on the island. The church is a central institution, shaping the rhythm of the workweek that ends with *to'ona'i*, Sunday lunch shared with family.[2] Saturdays are spent preparing for Sunday – shopping, cooking, sometimes preparing for special events at church. *Matai*, titled family leaders who manage family and village affairs through their political meetings, the *fono*, are as influential in urban areas as in the rural – calling on families when their support is needed.[3] In fact, the urban area is crowded with stores selling items specifically for *fa'alavelave* like pandanus mats, cases of frozen meat or tinned fish, as well as soda and crackers (see figure 6.2).

Fa'alavelave are ritualized events organized around significant life markers such as weddings and funerals. Driving through the island, you can spot fa'alavelave by the rows of chairs shaded by large white tents that fill the grassy spaces at the center of villages. Events like fa'alavelave have made Pacific Islands communities places anthropologists have long studied to learn how foodways, social hierarchies, and kinship connect.[4]

Plantations – the small plots of land worked by families – supply taro, breadfruit, and bananas, among other things, for daily consumption and for fa'alavelave. These are also spaces where families can keep pigs or chickens and grow fruit like papaya. Maintained on customary land, plantations are also an important cultural and political symbol of fa'asamoa. Yet people bemoan that youth don't want to work them anymore. They want to work for money, migrate, or go to a university. Men who still maintain plantations describe this work as an essential part of their identity, as Afu, a man in his sixties, did when he described himself as a farmer. His wife, who Jessica also interviewed, was in a leadership position in the government. This couple was proud to have, what they would call, "the best of both worlds," as she worked and earned a salary allowing them some comforts, and he maintained gardens so they could eat starches every day and enhance their meals with dishes like chicken soup with leafy greens.

Samoan foodscapes have changed dramatically in the past seventy-five years.[5] Diets once rich in fish, fruit, and root crops have changed to include highly processed foods like rice, noodles, and tinned fish.[6] As a result of this changing foodscape – likely compounded with daily stressors related to increasing inequalities wrought by globalization and changing labor patterns – Pacific Islands like Samoa bear a high burden of obesity. The World Bank estimates that 70 per cent or more of all deaths in the Pacific Islands are related in some fashion to non-communicable diseases.[7] Of all the regions in the world, Oceania – that is, a region that spans the Pacific Ocean to include Australasia, Melanesia, Micronesia, and Polynesia – has had the greatest increase in average BMI between 1980 and 2010.[8] Recent statistics suggest that over two-thirds of the adult Samoan population are obese. This is twice the rate in the United States and almost twentyfold the rate in Japan.[9] Perhaps not surprisingly, addressing obesity and the chronic diseases like diabetes associated with it have emerged at the center of most health interventions in Samoa.

Most of these health promotion efforts have been focused on changing individual eating habits, and encouraging consumption of more locally grown fruits and vegetables. Diet-related posters hang in clinics, differentiating the unhealthy (processed imported foods) from the healthy alternatives.[10] While the clinics also post ideal weight charts designed for Pacific Islanders, other posters are mostly taken directly from foreign public health campaigns. The National Health Promotion Policy similarly focuses on individual behavior with statements like this: "All individuals and communities in Samoa are enabled and supported to lead healthier lives through having control over their health and well-being, throughout their life-cycle," and the state is committed to a "nation-wide collaborative effort in achieving a common goal by encouraging all Samoans to have control over their health."[11] Though the policy focuses on creating supportive environments, multi-sectoral collaboration, and community action, the posters and other health materials clearly indicate weight loss as an individual endeavor – mostly by eating differently.

WHY ARE PEOPLE FAT? "THE WHOLE FAMILY IS RESPONSIBLE"

"It's their fault," Katerina (aged twenty-three) explained emphatically. People's bodies are their own responsibility. "Every time, I would say [it's] their fault." When people get fat, it is because of their own actions, she said, adding: "I would say typical Samoan eating, typical Samoan food, getting the typical Samoan body. Because they grew up in families, they don't have a liberal education. They feel this food is the best food. This is just how it is. Everybody eats this food. The cycle continues." This last statement belies a more complex Samoan explanation. Yes, people are responsible for their bodies, but they are also subject to powerful social and political forces that sustain certain ways of eating. Time after time people would say to Jessica that individuals are responsible. Usually, this would be followed by a "but ..." What could they afford? Really, the whole family was responsible. This is not surprising in the context of Samoa where family connection and mutual support are at the core of individual identity.

Given this strong Samoan emphasis on family, it is initially surprising that laziness (*paiē*) was cited as the culprit for fatness and diabetes. But this discourse of laziness circulated widely, from informal conversations with health-care providers to the daily newspaper, the *Samoa Observer*. Prime Minister Tuilaepa Aiono Sailele Malielegaoi said:

> There are plenty of mangoes, pawpaws, bananas and bread-fruit falling off and rotting on the ground, plenty of fish in the sea. The problem is too many people are coming into

> town and loafing around. They are lazy and do not want to
> go back to their village to work the land. They should stay in
> their village where their lands are and develop it.

Tuilaepa continued, some "Samoans think that not having a car, a TV or a European house is poverty. Those are luxuries. Having none of those is certainly not poverty."[12] The prime minister's comments generated a lot of discussion in Samoa about who can determine what is a luxury and what is a necessity.

This basic idea, shared by many, suggests that responsibility and blame cannot be assigned without attention to its multiple levels of context. On the first level are the household, the village, the church; on the next level is the nation; and finally, on the third level are global food trade and transnational migration. Laziness was thus articulated at multiple levels to express ambiguities that arose around changing food norms and rising inequalities. Tausa, a woman in her sixties who had lived in both the United States and Asia, explained that Samoa had changed since she was a girl. "The lifestyles have really changed," she explained. "People are lazy. We're not working as hard. I talk to a lot of people who are younger than us, and as soon as you're fifty, they think you're old, so they don't do this or that – it's ridiculous. It's all about your attitude." She bemoaned how men and women seemed to be dying in their forties. "What prevents this generation from making a change?" Jessica asked. Tausa responded pointedly, "Laziness and attitude." Health requires effort, she continued. "You need to work at it. You need to also reduce." Like Katerina, she conjured an image of "a typical village family" that she thought would probably eat "whatever's available today." If they could avoid it, she felt, they would avoid going fishing or working on the planation. "It's all about attitudes."

Princess (age thirty-six), a pseudonym she chose herself, said of her brothers, "They just don't have a heart for plantation work." In other words, they were not motivated like her father was, even though they were raised going to the plantation every weekend. Others explained more pragmatically: if you worked in town, then you could pay someone else to work the plantation. For some, this could be slightly shameful. It revealed that one had enough money to pay other people *and* that there weren't any family members who were willing to work the land for the benefit of the family.

This simultaneous tension between the family plantation and the realities of urban life made it difficult for interviewees to say the individual was fully and completely responsible for their weight. Even Katerina said boldly, "The whole family is responsible, especially for the upbringing of the kids to become healthy human beings." In other words, the typical Samoan body she described developed because of the environment of the family. Individuals were responsible insofar as they were able to make decisions within their families – children could not be held responsible.

Families were thus the focus of discussions about responsibilities because multiple forms of social and economic change impacted them as a unit. First, there was the "the money factor," explained Kilisi. She was willing to cut vegetables from her diet, eating only rice and meat, for example, if that meant there was more food for the whole household. But, she said, "at the end of the day, it's down to the person. If you want it that bad, you can do it." So, people were left to figure out how to create change they wanted but felt constrained at every turn because "everything cost money now," Kilisi's husband would say, especially if you lived in town where you most likely had to purchase all your foods. This was convenient, as you didn't have to grow food yourself or pay someone else to do it – but it meant your choices were limited by your budget.

The role of the cost of food was also a source of disagreement. Vegetables, which stood in for having a healthy diet, were considered both expensive and cheap. They were expensive because they needed to be purchased. Local varieties, though, didn't cost much. Most people could recall a time in their life when they didn't spend money for food, or at least only spent money on what were considered staples – tea, sugar, bread, and meat. Vegetables, in contrast, were not seen as staples. But through health promotion, most Samoans now associate vegetables with health and agree they *should* be staples. Some felt this new requirement, an added expense, was onerous. Katerina, who works for the Samoan government, said, "Good stuff is so expensive. We can't just tell people to eat healthy and healthy food is not accessible." The government, through public health efforts, tells citizens that they must "eat the rainbow" to reduce obesity and related diseases. But, the government, she indicated, wasn't acting responsibly to ensure that "there are healthy options available." Chicken was particularly problematic. Why were the imported frozen chickens purchased at the store so fatty? Why was this fatty meat so cheap? Local fresh chickens were skinnier, but not widely available in markets. Cheap meat was not healthy; it was potentially "poisonous," yet it was viewed as a required staple.[13] "There's no choice" said Lili (age sixty-eight), because other meats were far more expensive.

Some Jessica interviewed, however, felt the opposite. Eating unhealthy imported foods was expensive and left you hungry. Cheeseburgers at McDonald's, a luxury item, were so small that you would have to eat multiple burgers to feel full. Rice and chicken were filling, but more expensive than locally produced fruits, vegetables, and starches like taro – even if you didn't grow them yourselves. Pua (age fifty-one) felt particularly strongly about this. She had gone through a significant health transformation that began with a Polynesian Zumba group. The mostly women's group would meet at lunchtime, so she would skip lunch and dance, and sweat with a group of twenty to fifty women from 12 noon to 1 p.m. every day.

The midday heat made sweating as normal as drinking water. What Jessica remembered most about the classes was the comradery. Friends greeted one another and complemented each other on their *puletasi* (Samoan-made clothing, tailored for the individual). New people were welcomed. As quickly as the women arrived and changed their clothing, they rushed into the cramped locker room after class. It would be packed with women of all sizes, some white women, some Samoan, busily showering, changing, pulling back long hair into large buns that sat on the crown of their heads. The room quickly changed in smell from the sweat of a hard workout to perfumed lotion and deodorants as the women hurriedly jumped back into their cars – usually carpooling – to get back to their offices. And then the gym was empty. It was 5 p.m. before the same routine started again. The carpool created a kind of accountability, as people saved time (from walking) or money (from having to take a taxi). In large government buildings, where multiple offices were housed, you could ride the elevator to pick up friends. Facebook was another space where workout plans were solidified and complimented, the women sharing how proud they were of each other and challenging friends to keep going.

When I asked Pua why the Zumba group helped her prioritize her health, she said, "I felt that's where I belonged at the time." Now,

Pua owns her own gym, on the second floor of a crisply painted commercial building. From the street you can see the exercise equipment or classes doing circuit training through the opened glass doors that extended the workout space onto the balcony. The experiences Pua collected during her Zumba days inspired her to think creatively about building her own business. She said, "I love the feeling that I get just seeing somebody else enjoying the exercise and walking out of the building feeling so good about themselves. That, to me, is very rewarding. It makes me feel good." Pua also aimed to help people by asking them about their eating; she tells them it's simple. Just cut the soda, cut the sweets, cut the bread and rice. Eat the veggies and the meat but be sure to cut the fat off.

Others, notably also in the fitness industry, said there needed to be more education on how to prepare cheap meat. Amosa (age thirty-eight) was adamant about this. He mentioned several times that double-boiling meat was a great way to reduce fat consumption. When he moved back to Samoa from New Zealand, he was shocked that his schoolmates, who were now grown men, had become so fat. He moved in with his family while his house was being built. During this time, he was "disgusted" by the chicken. Not only did the family not trim the fat, they didn't boil it first before preparing it in the main dishes. This explained, he said, "the size of our people here." His wife also reflected on the difficulties of moving back in with family, a household of sixteen people, after living as a nuclear family for many years in New Zealand. The kids ate more noodles than she liked, and a lot more bread. She felt she couldn't say anything outright, but "slowly," she said, "we just sort of had to, um, not train, but kind of make suggestions that, you know, maybe boil the chicken twice and remove the oil, and um – use spices, and try and get some more vegetables. So, we – we introduced at least vegetables in the diet."

Blame was thus again allocated at different scales; each interviewee would start by articulating individual responsibility but then expanded from there. Individuals had a responsibility to eat differently, to purchase food conscientiously, or to grow foods when they could. At the next level, the family had a responsibility to prioritize family spending on healthy foods or to subsidize the work of those who could work plantations. The family had a responsibility to create a nutritious environment for children, who would otherwise not be capable of future responsibility if this initial environment had not been provided. The government was the next level, which was responsible for creating trade and agricultural environments that made healthy foods available at affordable prices. The government was responsible for ensuring that the chicken procured through fair trade was indeed safe for consumption. The interviewees thus articulated complex explanations about what caused fatness. However, individual responsibility was entrenched, if only as a starting place for deeper discussion of who or what was to blame.

WHEN IS FAT BAD? "YOU'VE GOTTEN BIG!"

After the recorder had been turned off, Lanuola (twenty-seven) and Jessica continued eating their fish burgers – battered, fried fish with cabbage slaw topped with a thick dollop of mayonnaise. Jessica always ate it with the local hot sauce, with fries on the side. This day was no different, other than the awkwardness of the interview formalities, which was markedly different than how Jessica normally interacted with Lanuola, her former research assistant. Lanuola interviewed diabetes patients alongside Jessica and then transcribed, translated, and consulted on those interviews during previous research periods. Interviewing Lanuola was therefore a bit strange, but she obliged. At first, they stumbled clumsily through the pre-scheduled set of questions because Jessica already knew the answers. Where did you grow up? What about your education? Then they eased into it, as Lanuola talked about her own struggles with fat, with eating, and with friends teasing her about her weight gain since having a baby. When the interview was complete, and the recorder was off, Jessica asked what questions she missed – "what would you have added?" No new questions, though Lanuola giggled, "I'm glad I know you." "What do you mean?" Jessica asked. With a twinkle in her eye and eyebrows askew Lanuola replied, "I couldn't talk about this stuff to just anyone. If I didn't know you, I would have just said, yes, no, vegetables are good, obesity is bad." "Why is that, do you think?" Jessica asked. "Most Samoans, they think it's nice. There's sarcasm around the whole idea of trying to tell people to eat healthy. If you say, 'Oh, that's bad,' they'll say stuff like, 'Oh, we're all gonna die.' That kind of stuff." Across interviews, people talked about the humor involved when talking about fat, a humor that was ironic and cynical.

A question that Jessica's interviews often led into was, "Why is fat funny?" The first way to answer this question was to understand what a good body looks like. Interviewees would say: "A normal size. An average size. Not big, not too skinny. Moderate, medium build. You have to be in the middle." Kilisi would say, turning her head side to side, showing disapproval, "You can't win." The motivation to have a normal body size meant there was constant social attention focused on bodies that were too thin or too big and on people who exercised too much or too little or ate too much or too little. Each of these "too little" or "too much" categories could be made humorous. Most interviewees agreed that the most common way body size was addressed was through teasing. The most easily imagined scenario was picturing you had returned from travel, you see friends or family, they say, "You've gotten big!" Not a compliment, but not an insult, this kind of statement was more a way to show that you noticed the person and that their travel must have been good if they were able to become a little fatter. Alofa, a woman in her forties who worked as an educator at one of the universities, lightheartedly explained that if her auntie told her she looked beautiful, she'd ask, "What's wrong with you? How come you're not insulting me right now?" Commenting on fatness showed that she and her auntie were comfortable and close – "so close that I can make this stupid comment."

Humor and teasing were ways to express the two-meanings of fatness: fatness could index being cared for, but fatness was also associated with sickness as current public health campaigns were suggesting. When interviewees mentioned Pacific-specific ideal body charts, they also expressed ambivalence. People grappled with the fact that Samoans are, and have been, larger than others like white people or people from Asia. Yet sicknesses related to weight had only emerged recently. The stories here were efforts by urban Samoans to make sense of how fat, and the sicknesses that have come from rapid nutritional and social change, can have multiple meanings.

Similarly, when people commented on thinness, it was a way of showing care. Tausa explained that when she was a girl, the women in her village would call her *siama*, which translates as germs but generally refers to thinness that indicates sickness. They'd ask her if she was okay and ask her mother if she was sick. She wasn't. She had just always been small, and now in her sixties, she was still happily thin.

> They always joke. It was never meant to be a mean comment or down talking. I mean, now I understand. I think back over it and I laugh about it. I'm glad that they even had the time to be talking to me. I mean, obviously, they recognized, "Oh, she's so-and-so's daughter." At least they were talking to me.

In other words, this commentary on body size was a way to recognize her parents and her family. What else would they have to say to a child? Adults would otherwise ignore children, "You're just a kid. You don't get talked to. Remember, that's a fa'asamoa, too. There's no conversation with kids."

Others talked about how it was motivating when a person close to them teased them about their body size, though sometimes it would hurt. Malia (sixty-one) told a typical story. She felt you could be "big and healthy" if you "moved all the time." This was how she grew up, eating only two meals a day – meals made from foods that she and her family grew. She did household chores, keeping her body moving. When Malia moved to town when she was a young woman, this is when things changed, she said. She didn't have chores; she didn't keep a garden; and she hired a girl to clean their house. Her family started eating imported foods, though they always ate vegetables, she insisted. She went from feeling healthy (but big) to feeling heavy. She noticed she was sleeping all the time. She would get up to eat and return to bed. She felt herself getting bigger, her clothes weren't fitting. She hated herself. She would make excuses to avoid leaving the house. She felt depressed. She would slouch when she sat down, which her sisters began to comment on. One sister called her ugly in front of the whole family. She cried and started to pray, saying, "I know it hurts, but God show me the way to get over this." Her sister persisted, and when she asked her to stop making those comments, she said she wouldn't until Malia made a change. She started going to the gym, attending Zumba classes, cleaning the house herself, growing a garden, and "reducing" her food. Her sister stopped remarking on her body, only once saying, "Oh, you look different now."

Malia's story makes clear that fat was bad on multiple levels – physically, it made her tired; emotionally, it made her depressed; socially, it made her the object of unwanted attention. Emotional suffering was assumed to accompany an unhealthy large size as people said that when they saw very large people, they immediately felt sorry for them. They must not love themselves. They must be mocked. Even if they were high status, "I feel sorry for them." Yet each interviewee explained fat was normal. It was associated with high status, but fatness and high status went together now because these people didn't exercise and they ate a lot. Not necessarily because they were well cared for and strong, as was historically thought to be true. Now interviewees said it's normal to walk into a room and see mostly fat people.

Nearly every interviewee mentioned the prime minister as an example of how normal it was to be fat. He was fat and also powerful. Leadership or other high-status people were fat because they ate so much at events, from meetings to funerals. Tausa explained:

> Everything we do is measured by food. When you have a big function, the first thing that's wrong is, okay, you may have really good food, but if the portion is not big, your function is not good. It's got to be a huge serving of whatever. That's sad, 'cause you don't even look at the quality of the food, but you just look at the quantity.

When Tausa was a girl she remembered preparing for these kinds of functions, served buffet style so one could choose the portion. Baskets would be filled to bring food home to family. They always served a variety of seafood and raw fish. Nowadays, she felt "we are fighting with plastic and big hunks of frozen chicken," meaning people were competing by providing platters of food and cases of frozen meat at these functions. Tausa was irked by this, commenting, "The amount, I am always in awe of the amount of food people consume."

Despite this normalization of being fat, most interviewees iterated that it was more difficult for girls and women to be big. Women's bodies received more attention for being large, Katerina explained. When I asked what an ideal body size would be for a woman and a man she responded, "See, this is the funny thing. With couples, if men are big, fat," she paused and asked if she could even say "fat," which Jessica told her, "of course." "Okay. If the man is fat and the girl is skinny, it's sort of okay. At a wedding, nobody's gonna bash the man. But, if a skinny guy is with a fat woman, it's just a complete disaster." Her own brother had recently broken up with a girl because she wouldn't change her eating habits to lose weight.

Some women in their twenties and thirties feared having children, because they said this meant they would certainly (and permanently) gain weight. Having children came with a host of other responsibilities and limitations that were associated with that gain, including cooking and being tied to the house, unable to get out to do any physical activity. Young men, they noted, could spend time playing rugby, lifting weights, and dressing in sportswear that was form-fitting and with hair styled with care. Sina (age twenty-nine) laughingly explained how she found the young men in her church who were preparing for a dance competition crowded around a mirror trying to perfect their hair. This story was all the more hilarious, from her perspective, because they were preening in the weight room they had established in the church hall. She teased them, "Stop trying to be pretty!" From the women's perspective, young men focusing on their looks and crafting muscular bodies was frivolous. It was something to be done because they did not have serious obligations or limitations the ways young women did.

Thus, we see that fat was not seen as either strictly good or bad. Instead, movement and food mattered in creating healthy bodies, ones that could be fat and sick, or large and strong. People mulled over judgments and stereotypes, their own and others, and were thoughtfully aware of the contradictions that arose around the multiple meanings of fatness.

WHO IS FAT? "SAMOANS LOVE THEIR FOOD"

This was a common refrain uttered in interviews and throughout Jessica's research over the past ten years – often iterated as a first point of explanation for rising obesity and related diseases. Food was an essential part of fa'asamoa, but foods have dramatically changed, as has fa'asamoa. Jessica has written about this elsewhere – that culture is a quick explanation for the rapid rise in obesity and other related diseases across Oceania. Certainly, culture is often blamed for what are, in fact, symptoms of economic disparities.[14] When people went back and forth in conversations between focusing blame on the culture, the individual, or the economic context, they grappled with the complex and often interrelated factors that have changed everyday life in Samoa. Yes, food was an essential tool for expressing the complexities of respect, status, generosity, and kinship. It was a "beautiful part of the culture," as one interviewee would say, so as not to lay such blame. But the way this part of the culture was practiced today left many feeling that it was out of sync with the realities of daily life where office work dominated, food was expensive, and opportunities to grow food were limited.

This speed of change meant people were often struggling to articulate how fatness connected to personal identity and place in the community. Fatness was at the same time associated with power and status and also with poverty and ignorance. Fatness was normal, accepted, and also stigmatized. It was okay as long as one's body had a steady shape and was able to move. Fatness was stigmatized when it intersected with what was seen as laziness – whether from wealth or poverty, from too many luxuries or too much dependence on cheap, unhealthy foods. Thus, both the wealthy and the less wealthy could be fat, albeit with slightly different explanations given.

One way that people created differences based on fatness between people was by talking about race – as Loto did when he reminded me that Samoans are larger than white people, but still healthy. Alofa (forty-two) explained that her family always ate healthily, which helped her stay thin in her youth and then later shaped her own eating preferences. The family always ate vegetables, because she noted, "I am half Chinese," which she thought helped her "metabolism stay a little bit up." The Samoan side of her family, her father's family, would make fun of her for being small, in part because they never accepted her mother who came from a mixed Samoan–Chinese family. They would tease her about her small size, drawing attention to her different tastes in food. Others talked about making fun of palagi women as they exercised furiously at the gym. Katerina said: "It's always the skinniest girls going all out at the gym. So, you're like, 'Um, girl? What are you doing?'" Such fanatic health consciousness, which racializes food preferences and body size, was viewed as decidedly un-Samoan.

What was Samoan about health was returning to a balance in life that involved local foods – that were touted as organic, fresh, and natural – and physical activity either from exercise or chores. Exercise was incorporated into Samoan social life for urban women through Zumba or exercise classes where participants felt they were part of a community supporting each other to live well, or as they might say, "live clean." It wasn't just the exercise that kept the women coming, it was friendship and social support. When women were proud for not having help to tend to their house, or men proudly shared that they kept a small plantation behind their house, they were claiming social life as a healthy life. In each interview, people mentioned the "old days," a time when "the culture was easy, peaceful, and everything you get, everything comes from your hands. The work of your hands." This contrasts to today where "everyone can exist alone" or is "living beyond their means."

INTERVIEWING AND EATING IN APIA

The interviews for this book had to be in good, comfortable social contexts. This was impossible without some kind of food, and, in fact, most interviews took place over two shared meals. Most interviewees were working women who were pressed for time, the best time for them to meet Jessica was during their lunch break from work, or right after work had finished. They often only had an hour or so to spend with her before family responsibilities beckoned. For the first meeting, Jessica would buy coffee or tea – lattes, long blacks, English Breakfast tea – then for follow-up meetings she'd buy lunch or breakfast – usually grilled chicken sandwiches, fish burgers, or omelets.

Meeting in restaurants and lobbies was essential because it was nearly impossible to meet in people's homes. Visiting people's homes either meant you were part of the family, or more likely, you were a formal guest. As such, if you did visit someone at home, it was best not to tell them ahead of time as this would obligate them to provide generous foods to greet you with. If you did arrive unannounced, as would be preferred, food appeared but it didn't need to be as special.

Youth ran to shops to buy crackers or soda, while other household youth would quickly boil water for tea. Small tables would appear next to you, to provide a place to put your drinks. One of the clearest ways that Jessica learned how close she had become with her adopted family was when her partner visited, which was also the moment that she learned it's better to surprise than to announce a visit. When Jessica returned to the house with her partner, after church, she found a table elegantly dressed – with white table cloth and glassware she'd never seen – in the front sitting area of the house, a place where you could gaze out to the ocean peeking through the foliage of a giant mango tree. Within minutes, trays of food appeared. Not just the usual bananas (though they were there) but also taro, salads with artificial crab, oka, chicken, and sausages. Lemonade, not water. They ate with the elders, the youth and children waited. At the time, Jessica felt guilty that the family had gone to such effort and expense for her partner. Later, she realized how much she had become embedded in the household by virtue of the lack of fanfare she received when she shared meals with them, eating alongside the whole family together.

In Samoa, just as Jessica's own understandings of fat were shaped by her experiences of being embedded in a family, the meaning of fat in interviews emerged from listening to stories about family as well as money and urbanization. Growing disparities between those who live and work in the urban area and those who live in the rural areas and work plantations shape the meaning and experience of fatness. When we listen to these stories, the family is both vulnerable and responsible for the changing qualitiessssssssss of economic and social life. These stories show ambivalence about fat – it is both pitied and normalized. Those who identify as fat point to an environment where it seems impossible *not* to be fat. When the family is blamed, it is for not balancing cash-earning potential with support for those who grow and manage family plantations. This balance seems impossible to achieve as there were ever-increasing needs for cash and only very limited opportunities to earn it. Paying to maintain a plantation, or to purchase healthy food options were almost always the last priority. The stories here were efforts by urban Samoans to make sense of how fat, and the sicknesses that have come from rapid nutritional and social change, can have multiple meanings.

CHAPTER SEVEN

The Bigger Picture: Shared Beliefs about Fat

Our four-site study began with some basic questions about how our bodies are viewed in different societies. The themes we highlighted in writing the site-specific chapters addressed ideas about why people get fat, when fat is bad, and who gets fat. In each of our sites, people expressed their thoughts and experiences as to why people get fat. In general, there was often quick consensus that individuals were responsible for their fat, but, as people told us more about how they constructed individual responsibility, different notions of community became visible in the stories. In other words, individuals *did* claim responsibility for being fat but they also explained the ways that other (often structural) aspects of life prohibited them from making changes. Likewise, there was general belief across the sites that fat was bad, but the negative values ascribed to fat were neither monolithic nor static. Indeed, people in the sites spent considerable time recounting why fat was bad in specific kinds of contexts. These contexts varied across the sites, demonstrating the particularities of each field site. In trying to understand who was fat, according to the people we interviewed, we noticed that across the sites, interviewees could easily tell us who was fat, or likely to become fat. That is, people in Japan, the United States, Paraguay, and Samoa had expectations about what kinds of people are fat and how they might behave.

In this chapter, we look more closely at what people told us from a cross-cultural perspective. We identify meta-themes that make audible how people in each of the sites understood and experienced fat in their daily lives. Comparative ethnography highlights the internal logic of the ways that people in one place think about body weight, size, and health vis-à-vis other places. Meta-themes are a key means of accessing these internal logics. As we analyzed what our participants told us, six meta-themes emerged that resonated across all sites. This chapter is organized around the six emergent meta-themes, which are:

1. fat is one's own fault,
2. fat is a social failure,
3. fat is unhealthy,
4. fat is harder for women,
5. fat is an outcome of structural shifts, and
6. fat marks insider/outsider status.

Important distinctions within these six meta-themes did emerge again and again within and between the sites. In other words, they were neither monolithic nor static.

In this next step of systematic comparison, each of us chose typical exemplars that best represent how the meta-themes were expressed in the interviews at each site. "Typical exemplars" are direct quotes from one person that do a good job of capturing the essence of what many respondents were saying consistently, even if they were saying it in different words. To identify typical exemplars, we always work in the original language of the interviews; crucial social and cultural information gets lost even in the most careful translations. For each site, we then selected one interview quote that could be considered the most representative of each theme in each site. At this point, Cindi translated her exemplars from Japanese to English, Amber translated hers from Spanish (or Jopara) to English, and Jessica translated hers fully to English (her interviews were conducted in a mix of Samoan and English). Then, together, we finalized the list of typical exemplars that best highlighted the key differences and commonalities across the sites. Presenting these in people's own (albeit often translated) words – either here or in earlier chapters – gives the reader a further window into the different worldviews emerging from the data in each site.

While we describe these techniques, first in chapter 2 and now here, as analytically distinct stages, in reality there was much discussion, reiteration, and rethinking at each stage of analysis among the five of us. For example, we often discussed our thematic and meta-thematic findings as a group: analyzing detailed descriptions from our interviews, integrating our analyses of meta-themes, and considering how each meta-theme manifested in each of the four site-specific datasets. We often had side discussions, in which we explored our own understandings of our data – for instance, were things that seemed culturally distinct really more similar cross-culturally than we had realized? And, of course, we read and commented on each other's analyses. Constant feedback from co-authors who understood the phenomena but not the context forced us to explain (and, often, rethink) our interpretations in productive ways.

CROSS-SITE META-THEME #1: FAT IS ONE'S OWN FAULT

Our detailing of cultural views shows that people across all the sites linked weight gains to people's own eating patterns, various stressors, costs, and personal responsibility. The changes in body weights were seen as broad, profound, and part of an irreversible process related to changing food environments. Running alongside the idea of macro-level change in people's ways of life, however, was the persistent notion that people are themselves to blame for their own weight and that solutions for excess weight rest on the individual. We have discussed this theme extensively in previous chapters, but briefly revisit it here.

People in all four sites tended to express that they experienced their own fat as their own failing, either as a result of a lack of self-control or some sort of moral fault. Consequently, people viewed others' large bodies as similar failures. Rosa, a sixty-year-old woman from Encarnación, told Amber: "It depends on each person's will and perseverance. My parents or my friends can tell me, 'Look, you have to lose weight: lose weight.' But if I don't take it seriously, I'll just continue at the same weight. It depends on each person, each person's own will." Rosa relied on a framework of personal blame to explain why she and others remained overweight. Likewise, in Apia, participants pointed out people were fat in a context of changing foodways because they were too lazy to grow their own food or prepare foods that took time and instead relied on convenience foods like canned meats, frozen (sometimes fried) chicken, or rice that could be bought in the stores. In Osaka, interviewees explained that the demands of work environments encroached on any time to be healthy but talked about the blame for their own weight as being squarely placed on what they ate or how little they exercised. In north Georgia, respondents also lamented the loss of traditional foodways and generational change in what, how, and with whom people eat. Some saw this as part of the broader processes that led to weight gain. Most nonetheless said they felt that the work of controlling weight still rested entirely with the individual, most particularly in the need for disciplined approaches to self-restricted eating.

CROSS-SITE META-THEME #2: FAT IS A SOCIAL FAILURE

The comparison across the sites also shows that people typically identified fat with failure. This is because shared social meanings ascribed to fat facilitated the devaluing of people who are fat, in combination with theme one's shared social meaning that ascribed blame for fat to individuals. Fat stigma could take the form of self-shaming or of others engaging in shaming behavior directed outwards. Again, these stigmatizing behaviors were discussed in all of the sites. Disgust or mocking, either self-directed or projected by others (in or out of one's own network), was managed in a variety of ways, showing great diversity depending on place, time, and who was involved.

In Osaka, fat shaming manifested most strongly in references to someone as *fuketsu-na*, which means a person is dirty due to their own moral failings. In this reference, fat people, especially overweight men, were imagined as sweaty and oily; in this way, they were also described as a nuisance. That is, by drawing attention to themselves, they were viewed as an inconvenience to others, as well as faintly disgusting.

In contrast to body odor, in north Georgia, Encarnación, and Apia, the role of clothes was mentioned as a point of shame. In Apia, for example, people talked about feeling shame when their clothes became too tight. Wanting to cover up flesh perceived as excessive was a theme for people in north Georgia. In Encarnación, people also reported feeling shame for ill-fitting clothes, and said that they expected to be ridiculed. For example, twenty-nine-year-old Estefanía told Amber: "I have a friend … She is quite old: thirty-six years old and can't have a child because she does not want to have a boyfriend. And why does she not want to have a boyfriend? Because she's self-conscious about her body. And she sometimes cries because we don't go out, because nothing looks good on her." The friend was self-conscious because she felt she was too fat. Not looking good in clothes and feeling shame about one's body were frequently articulated reasons why people in Encarnación would avoid attending social functions like parties, which in turn directly affected the health of their social networks.

Perceived failure due to fatness was thus intertwined with fat shaming in all four locations but the ways in which fat shaming manifested, and the power of this shaming, could be very different. In Apia, people said that they commonly joked about fat, especially with close family members, as a way to express care by noticing that a person's body had changed. For example, forty-two-year-old Alofa told Jessica: "[If my aunt told me I was beautiful] I'll be like, 'What's wrong with you? How come you're not insulting me right now?'" At other times, joking was experienced as more shaming but was still thought to help the person being shamed see the need for change. In other words, it was still seen as constructive. In Encarnación, too, overt public joking about weight was generally socially acceptable and considered a suitable reaction to someone being overweight, including in the ways people interacted within the family.

In Osaka, discussions of fat people in general and overt (rude) examples of fat shaming in particular were shied away from by most interviewees and a similar attitude prevailed in north Georgia. The exception was within the family, a space where fat shaming was reported as a common occurrence by all the Japanese participants and many of the US participants. Cindi heard many stories like thirty-eight-year-old Junko's: "My brother used to tell me that I had 'sausage arms' or he'd say: 'If you lost a bit of weight you'd be so cute.'" The chapter focused on north Georgia already includes a lengthy quote from Christina, who told Sarah that her family was fat but also routinely stigmatized fatness and fat people as lazy welfare recipients. Another participant, Amy, also quoted in the north Georgia chapter, described in detail her parents shaming her throughout her childhood for her weight because they were so worried it would negatively affect her social mobility. Public politeness and private stigma thus collided in the Japanese and US sites.

One interesting aspect of the cross-cultural comparison around this theme is that joking, verbalized shaming, and individual weight being read as social failure did appear across all four sites but the shame and stigma were stronger in the sites that were more careful in how they spoke about fat. In other words – and echoing an observation we made about Paraguay in the introduction – people in Apia and Encarnación reported much more explicit experiences of being told they were fat and looked terrible but were less likely to report being upset and bothered about these experiences. In contrast, people in north Georgia and Osaka generally reported more veiled stigma experiences – especially in adults and especially outside the family – but were more likely to feel stigmatized and unhappy as a result. Our interpretation (others are possible) is that the larger national context in each place matters in how people interpret teasing that equates fat with failure. If, as in Osaka, the social consequences of fatness truly are dire, then the teasing is taken seriously; if, as in Apia, the social consequences of fatness are more mixed, then the teasing is taken more lightheartedly.

CROSS-SITE META-THEME #3: FAT IS UNHEALTHY

People across the sites also collectively connected fat – and more specifically, Obesity – to physical illnesses. This is not surprising when one considers the anti-Obesity campaigns that have been conducted in each place, campaigns that have stressed the elevated risk for diabetes, joint pain, asthma, sleep apnea, high blood pressure, hypertension, and cardiovascular disease that comes with higher weight. Slippery connections were also made between higher weight and emotional instability, bolstered by the attitudes of failure and individual responsibility outlined above. On the other hand, the degree to which people believed fat equaled disease did differ across the sites.

People with large bodies could mitigate certain judgments through specific behaviors. For example, in Osaka, interviewees explicitly noted that cheerful, energetic, and clean fat people were not viewed as being as unhealthy as fat people who sweated visibly and appeared lazy. In north Georgia, the importance of eating healthily – not visiting fast food restaurants regularly, not consuming massive amounts of soda, refraining from eating fried foods and carbohydrates – was also highlighted by many participants as an important behavior for people judged to be overweight or obese. Significantly, negative judgments were not completely eliminated through "good fatty" displays of cheery self-discipline,[1] and the conflation of fatness with ill health was particularly resistant to mitigating behaviors. By this, we mean that a fat body was seen as more likely to be diseased, regardless of how cheerful and good tempered the person was, how strenuously they dieted, how many gyms they visited, and so on.

For many of the people we talked to, unhealthy Obese bodies were characterized by medical numbers (e.g., resting blood glucose numbers or blood pressure) or by the physical illnesses that global public health has taught populations to associate with larger bodies. Mia, a thirty-five-year-old woman in Encarnación, noted that "hypertension, diabetes, circulatory diseases, cholesterol, triglycerides, joint pain ... I have it in my family. My grandmother had diabetes, hypertension. Another one: my grandfather had heart problems but he was also overweight and all that ... My dad, for example, died of diabetes. So you see how it is." Likewise, in north Georgia, Rosemary (a woman in her sixties) told Sarah, "I'm technically diabetic, although I don't take medication ... And I've been able to control it with diet ... Definitely, weight is associated with it ... It would be healthy if I could lose fifty pounds. I mean, I know that." In Apia, people linked fat to metabolic diseases such as diabetes and to mortality. Twenty-nine-year-old Sina told Jessica, "Everybody else is getting it [diabetes] earlier or dying early ... People dying in their thirties and forties. I was telling my class. I'm like, we should be concerned." In Apia, people linked other ailments to fat as well, including breathing difficulties, limited mobility, listlessness, and other cardiometabolic illnesses. Men were described as especially at risk. People in Osaka told Cindi similar stories: according to sixty-three-year-old Kikue, her husband and son complained about "aches and pains, in their hips, back and knees," and Kikue further declared that "my husband is overweight and my son is chubby, but they don't really move around much."

Understandings of these diseases, their connections with body size and weight, and what they looked like in people's everyday lives were where the cultural differences emerged across the sites. Thus, in the Samoan site, a fat person who had visible difficulty breathing, struggled with diabetes, and experienced mobility issues had an unhealthy body, but a body of equivalent size with no accompanying visible and experienced problems would not necessarily be read the same. When comparing across the sites, the strongest ideas about fat being unhealthy emerged in the north Georgia and Osaka sites. For example, in Osaka, people talked at length about their "concern" for people who they perceived to be fat. The effects of the *metabo* law will likely also be profound in reinforcing people's ideas that a bigger girth leads to disease. Similarly, in north Georgia, people's views reflected classic public health messaging about Obesity, possibly a side effect of many recent campaigns within the state of Georgia to reduce Obesity rates. Most of the women who were in their early twenties at the time they were interviewed, for example, told Sarah that they had their BMIs collected regularly in physical education classes in public high school, and one participant went on to explain that her (male, middle-aged) physical education teacher spoke with her, giving her eating and exercise advice, after her BMI measurement put her in the Overweight category. By contrast, fat was viewed much more relationally and flexibly by people in both the Samoan and Paraguayan sites.

CROSS-SITE META-THEME #4: FAT IS HARDER FOR WOMEN

Our analysis indicates that dealing with fat was socially more difficult for women in all sites, even in places where men were viewed as more at risk of becoming Obese. In all sites, women seemed to worry more about their bodies and worked more to control their food intake or exercise to lose weight. In all sites, the social consequences of having a large body – being seen as unattractive, unhealthy, lazy, unworthy of work promotions or romantic interest, and so forth – were paid more heavily by women than by men. For example, in Osaka, thirty-eight-year-old Hanako told Cindi: "Women should be thin and pretty, like a celebrity. Not men, it's different for them. Like my husband, he drinks all the time and is out of shape [and it's fine]." This idea that men could have "beer bellies" (*biruppara*) and still be viewed as fitting within a social norm was a point of discussion for many Japanese women that Cindi interviewed. Likewise, twenty-three-year-old Katrina, one of the Samoan site's participants, told Jessica, "If the man is fat and the girl is skinny, it's sort of okay. At the wedding, nobody's just gonna bash the man. If a skinny guy is with a fat woman, it's just a complete disaster." In this way, women were required to attend more to their body shape and size. For men across the field sites, a large body could signal and symbolize more than just being overweight and a lack of exercise. That is, larger male bodies could be seen as unhealthy and disgusting by one person and as powerful by another, whereas women's fat bodies were far more likely to be viewed only as unhealthy and disgusting. This was put very succinctly by one of the participants in north Georgia. As already mentioned in the chapter focused on Georgia, Anna, who was in her early twenties, told Sarah: "It's okay to be that way if you're a big guy – a white male. You can throw your weight around ... metaphorically, but also literally." Many other people interviewed in north Georgia agreed that women faced more severe social judgments connected to their weight. Some of the women had thoughts about the unfair social acceptability of beer bellies in men in north Georgia that echoed those of the women in Osaka.

However, men were not immune to unrealistic body ideals and pressures to diet. In Osaka, men complained of weight gain, especially after marriage, and often stated that they needed to lose some weight. One of the men participants in north Georgia also talked about pressure from family members to lose or maintain a particular weight through exercise and dieting. Others talked about the pressure they put on themselves to maintain physical fitness. In Apia, young men were concerned with developing an athletic, "rugby body" and were permitted leisure time and socially acceptable independence to participate in those kinds of activities. As Samoan men aged, their large bodies were viewed as more acceptable as a sign of status and age, whereas women continued to feel pressure to stay thin as they aged.

Lastly, in all sites, family meals and maintaining children's healthy weights were seen as more women's work than men's work. Japanese women who were also mothers told Cindi about the pressure they felt to feed their children a variety of nutritional foods, not only to make sure that the children consumed healthy meals but also so that they developed their palettes. Only one Japanese man talked about helping with meal preparation (on Saturdays when he was not at work). In Encarnación and north Georgia, on the other hand, men talked about helping out with grocery shopping and meal preparation, including cooking. Relatedly, they talked about the shifting roles for men at home, including in the kitchen. In their grandparents' generation, the participants in Encarnación and north Georgia explained that men were rarely allowed in the kitchen, but nowadays, men could help with meal preparation and cooking. Nevertheless, in Encarnación, although people acknowledged that men assisted in the meal planning and preparation, meeting the family's nutritional needs was seen more as women's work.

CROSS-SITE META-THEME #5: FAT IS AN OUTCOME OF STRUCTURAL SHIFTS

We have said repeatedly in this book that a core contradiction across the interview data was people's recognition that changes in the global political economy, in combination with how this has affected particular communities (especially marginalized communities), have driven weight increases but their core belief continued to be that weight was still a personal responsibility. Our first cross-site meta-theme focused on the core belief of responsibility but the theme of changes to our larger environment affecting our everyday lives remained important. People of various ages across the sites reported that fat was a consequence of structural changes in food costs and availabilities, as well as in family and work culture.

Changes in the cost and availability of different foods, combined with perceived lack of time to prepare meals "from scratch" due to work, led to people eating and feeding their families differently. Most participants across the four sites noted this. As twenty-year-old university student Coleen told Sarah, "I would say [socioeconomic status is the big driver of weight gain and chronic disease] worldwide. Just because it seems like really nutrient-rich food is becoming more expensive or having access to it is more difficult ... Living in food deserts makes it hard to access [healthy food]." Here Coleen points out that the high cost of nutritious foods made it difficult for many people to be healthy, recognizing the link between poverty and weight that scholars have often discussed.[2] Most of the other participants in north Georgia also made connections between poverty, less buying power, and the fact that fewer people than ever before could "do for themselves" when it came to growing and cooking their own food. Similarly, in Encarnación, thirty-five-year-old Mia said, "It is much cheaper to go buy four empanadas than making a salad." In Osaka, thirty-two-year-old Hikari told Cindi that when they visit her parents (in another city), "they feed us fruits. My parents are a bit extravagant. But, for me and my husband, we are both working as hard as we can. Money is important. Our kids will need so much more [money] as they get older; fruit is really expensive, so if I give them dessert, it's ice cream ... we don't eat fruit very often." Due to their cost, fruits were seen as expensive even though they were the dessert preferred by many Japanese families.

In Paraguay, the changes in food were directly linked to lack of time as well as expense and these were further connected to non-healthy meals. Rosa, a sixty-year-old woman in Encarnación, told Amber, "Before, traditionally, our mother cooked Paraguayan foods and all that, boiling for four hours. A healthy food. Nowadays, maybe because of the work bustle, well, they cook a quick pan fry with a salad – that's it – or hamburgers, or fast food." The ability to take time to cook healthy foods combined with the high cost of such ingredients led to reliance on fast foods like hamburgers. Likewise in Encarnación, Estefanía (a twenty-nine-year-old woman) explained to Amber that she "started work before 7 [a.m.], and there wasn't time for breakfast ... on the road, I'd go buy a sandwich, juice or soda ... and go to work ... I think that's why I was eating so much junk food – because there was no time."

Changes to work culture were also implicated in these structural changes – and these changes affected not just the working person but their families as well. As Estefanía noted above, the reason she had no time was because of her job. As Tausa, a sixty-six-year-old woman in Apia, told Jessica,

> [People get fat] who do office work, hardly working plantations, cutting crops, and all those normal chores at work, like choppin' fire wood. I think those are the people that they always gaining weight. Well, you know, part of that is not just

the physical. It's also the mental stress. Because of the pile of work, the demands on you. Then I stay up so late and then I wake up early because I do all the ironing in my household. You know, I'm thinking it's not balancing the rest that you need.

Tausa recognized that new types of employment took a toll not just on the body but also psychosocially, with stress compounding due to housework and non-work obligations. In Japan similar stories were told. Many Japanese women talked about the work culture of their husbands who were company men. Specifically, the long days meant many men did not eat breakfast at all, had unhealthy lunches, and often had to go out for lavish company dinners. Hitomi, a thirty-one-year-old woman in Osaka, believed that "the stress of a company job contributes to heart disease" because of the poor eating habits that work demanded.

CROSS-SITE META-THEME #6: FAT MARKS INSIDER/ OUTSIDER STATUS

Across all sites, there was some articulated understanding that weight was a marker of being a social insider or outsider. This is a very complex concept and meta-theme to compare cross-culturally, because every society has distinct intersecting social categories, based on class, race/ ethnicity/nationality, place of employment, birthplace, education, and so on. People can simultaneously belong to certain groups in certain ways, while being considered outsiders in other ways (think of the difference between a religious identity and a national identity, for example). Further complicating the picture with respect to weight specifically is the fact that many people reported different ideas about weight and outsider status – sometimes, the same person even reported seemingly contradictory ideas about weight and insider/outsider status.

In most sites, fat was seen as a marker of who belonged to a certain class or socioeconomic status. Significantly, though, fat could mark belonging to upper or lower classes, depending on the site. In the American South, for example, fat was often viewed to be a marker of poverty, lack of education, or low social status. In the abstract, this combination (fat, ignorant, and poor) tended to be spoken of as characteristic of others/outsiders nearby – other communities and families within the same region. Complicating this framing, however, was the fact that most people with whom Alex and Sarah spoke either considered themselves fat or had friends and family who they considered fat – and people hesitated to equate fatness with lack of education and low status in these personal, known instances. In the Samoan and Paraguayan field sites, in contrast, it was wealthy people's fatness that was considered an outlier and "not fitting" the cultural norm. This was because wealthy people were seen as the ones having the means and food access to get fat, while poorer people struggled to get enough of the right kinds of foods. In the Samoan and Paraguayan field sites, literal overconsumption of resources – embodied on familial and individual bodies as fatness – was viewed negatively because those resources should be shared by the community. As Samoan participant Amosa, a thirty-eight-year-old man, told Jessica, "[Pastors are always fat.] Because they receive food. I'm saying, you know, they are getting the food free actually and perhaps the money too … You see a lot of poor people, you know, different people. You see our people, the way they look, sitting here [on the street], and then you see pastors, because you can tell by the way they're dressing. So that's [why] they are *lapo'a* [big] … He's big like that because he is a pastor."

Ideas about national predispositions toward fat made this concept even more complex. In north Georgia, and despite what we just said about fat marking lack of education and poverty in *others*, being fat was typically seen as a condition to which any Southerner was potentially susceptible. Jennifer, a woman in her fifties, told Sarah, "I think in the South there're probably two extremes. I think there's what we would consider the redneck, white trash trailer-park woman with her cigarette in her hand and just hugely obese … And then I think there's the more modern Southern woman, who is more conscientious and is more aware of her fitness and her health … And I think we, probably in the South, a lotta people tend to see that woman, the trailer-park woman, in their head." What Jennifer is getting at here is the idea that in fact, fat (and its associated trailer-park) looms as a possibility further down the road for many people she knows, regardless of how fit, educated, and financially stable they currently are. This meant that being fat was simultaneously talked about as a trait embodied by others and as a trait that any Southerner could be susceptible to. Moreover, susceptibility wasn't just perceived to be regional but also national. In the chapter focused on north Georgia, we commented that many people talked to us about the idea that the United States is problematically fat. The United States of Fat, we said. At the level of the nation, therefore, fat was portrayed as marking insider status (albeit, an unwanted one) for many people in our site in the United States.

Significantly, some interviewees in our other field sites agreed with this assessment of fat in the United States, but looking at it from outside. For participants in Osaka, this also mapped more generally onto their ideas about fat, white Westerners.

In Osaka, fat was seen as something that happened to non-Japanese people,[3] or, if it happened to Japanese people, it was due to them eating non-Japanese food. As Tomoko (a twenty-seven-year-old woman) noted: "Compared to Japanese people, French people are fat. They don't care if their bellies hang out or their belly button shows; French people are fatter than Japanese people." Tomoko went on to link this to her experience that French people have a high consumption of cheese and cream. Many participants connected Western foods, such as dairy products, fast food hamburgers and fries, with large non-Japanese bodies, linking eating fast food to fat, which then linked to outsider status. Indeed, nearly all of the participants in the Japanese site had either studied abroad (in Western countries) themselves or knew someone who did and they cited substantial weight gain during those times spent outside Japan. Many highlighted that people in the United States had particular issues with weight and fat.

In Apia, when a young Samoan person came back from time overseas and had put on weight, it could signify a lack of connection and not caring for family and tradition, thus placing that person in an outsider position. In the Samoa site, white people were considered smaller than Samoans. Additionally, people who expressed health consciousness, including a preference for vegetable consumption, were often viewed as outsiders. In the Paraguay site, Brazilians and Argentinians were identified as "fat others."

Taken together, the differences across the sites demonstrate that fat could be a marker of insider *or* outsider status, depending on social context. The sites demonstrate that the idea of cultural belonging, in contrast to "foreignness," could at times be linked closely with weight but was not solely determined *by* weight. The body is a complex site of everyday meaning-making, and the meanings a body accumulates depend on social context. Societies are always changing and shifting, and thus body weights and accompanying norms are also in flux.

CONCLUDING THOUGHTS

A cross-cultural research lens allows places and points of similarity and differences across the sites to be identified, investigated, and analyzed. The six cross-cutting themes found across all four sites have some important implications. A shared belief that a large body size can be modified based on an individual's will helps explain why many national and regional interventions for addressing Obesity around the globe continue to emphasize individual efforts, even as the current science suggests that, to be effective, the focus of such interventions should address the broader drivers such as a lack of investment in thoughtful urban planning or unrestrained multinational profit seeking. Japan and Samoa both have national health policies aimed at weight reduction or maintenance and reduction of metabolic diseases in general. Georgia has statewide programs as well. In each place, however, the policies are not having much of an effect on reducing people's weight or increasing their healthfulness. In the face of the enduring failure of these kinds of interventions and policies to lower weight and improve people's health, we have to ask why.

We look to these six cross-cutting themes as pointing to some of the ways in which people make sense of fat, eating, disease, and health to help us consider alternative ways to ensure people around the globe have access to nourishing environments. The overwhelming reports of individual responsibility, combined with the felt need to feed one's family nutritious, healthy meals, combined with daily negotiations around other felt needs and limitations, gets at the heart of the seemingly contradictory ways that people across sites negotiate their daily lives and family obligations. The overlapping reports that women bear the brunt of managing body size and weight for themselves and for their families underscores the ways in which women's lives across the sites have some fundamental similarities.

We'd be remiss, though, not to note that there are real differences between places that help to explain how the idea of individual responsibility has been taken up. In Samoa, while people expressed associations between laziness and fatness, it was usually in their capacities to care for others that their laziness was evaluated. This reflects the ways that the body in Samoa is more of a community achievement than an individual achievement and, ultimately, a community responsibility. When the body is considered a community achievement, individuals don't always consider it reasonable to have agency over their bodies in terms of the kinds of physical activity in which they engage or the kinds of care they might seek when sick. Similarly, in Paraguay, people often said their body size was their own personal responsibility when asked. However, their views on others' bodies were undergirded by a sense of communal care and responsibility for others. People repeatedly suggested that they had the responsibility to motivate family and friends to eat healthily, to extend offers to exercise together, and to create interpersonal relations in which healthy lifestyles were supported. In Paraguay, when people talked about their own failed personal responsibilities to be healthy, they framed them in terms of failures to invest time in community-building and to keep Paraguayan traditions of eating homemade healthy foods. People's tendencies to prioritize the temptations of contemporary life – fast food, sedentary days, even an overemphasis on physical bodies – were also seen by interviewees in Encarnación, to some extent, as a personal failure to engage with and support the Paraguayan community and values.

By contrast, in north Georgia, people articulated notions of individual responsibility and care for health and body that adhered more to classic neoliberal United States ideas. The basic unit interviewees focused on was typically the individual, not the family or the larger community. On the other hand, even in north Georgia, there were exceptions to this model: parents were held responsible for their children's health and bodies, for example. Moreover, distaste for fat laziness was at least partly rooted in articulated ideas of fat people failing to live up to notions that they would be productive members of society, instead serving as drains on community resources. Thus, even in the context of the United States, where individualized responsibility is extremely pervasive, the backdrop for any (fat-stigmatizing) discussion of social failure inevitably pulls in the collective.

The notion of individual responsibly in Osaka takes a particularly gendered tone. To say that Osakan people hold themselves individually responsible for their body weight and fat fails to account for the ways that women specifically are perceived to be the people who can and should keep themselves, their husbands, their families, and thus, the nation, healthy. These kinds of ideals or expectations are not surprising given that they were formally instituted at the national level in the early 1900s. Married women in particular expressed a deeply engrained sense in the interviews with Cindi that they must feed their families nutritious and highly varied foods so that their children's palates developed and their bodies grew appropriately. Osakan wives lamented that they were unable to feed their husbands healthy and nutritious foods due to busy work schedules and responsibilities – their husbands' work schedules made it difficult for them to fulfill their responsibilities. For Osakan men, work took precedence over showing up for nutritious family meals in terms of caring for the family. Financial stability trumped nutrition, in other words.

Nonetheless, the four sites illuminate how changing body sizes intersect with changing sociocultural norms and interlock with local contexts, values, and social structures. Our findings highlight that current global public health approaches to combating obesity are deeply embedded in cultural views about personal responsibility for weight. They also show that these approaches largely ignore the ways that body size may also signal social prestige, class, and belonging.

CHAPTER EIGHT

Conclusions: A Global Perspective on Weight

The so-called global epidemic of Obesity, and the ways in which it is viewed as a shifting pattern of global risk, can also be viewed as a cultural phenomenon, informed by very specific sociocultural perspectives.[1] For one thing, an attempt to understand the medical risks of weight based solely on body mass calculations and population-level data doesn't make much sense in view of what is happening to people in their daily lives and experiences. Furthermore, general public health advice about the need to control body weight sits at a confusing intersection of information about weight, bodies, food, and health that people encounter everywhere and must process continuously.[2] It defines the very problem itself in terms that actually offer little help to people – at least in terms of their own quests to live healthy and meaningful lives. Despite all that we know and understand about how such structural factors as power, political economy, environment, and epigenetics create certain kinds of risks for Obesity, the focus on individual responsibility plagues almost all weight interventions, both personal and professional.

It is clear that some people understand their body as a primary, inescapable, anchor. In Encarnación, north Georgia, and Osaka, the body figured prominently in defining a person, both as others saw them and as they saw themselves. In Apia, the body had less to do with perceptions of the individual self and more to do with the ways in which the body was seen as a social resource or a social liability.

In either case, however, informed by medical and other institutional efforts, people do embrace (to varying degrees) the idea that weight is an individual problem – their own problem. People repeatedly said that they feel that they should manage their diet and exercise and that they try to do so. Efforts at weight management by individuals, wherever they are, add to daily worries of lack of time, too much stress, or too little money. It's one of many things people are juggling.

What is perhaps one of the most surprising findings of our study is how aware people are that weight gain at the population or community level is a product of changing environments. Around the world, they consistently say that loss of traditional foodways, changing work demands, the busy-ness of contemporary life, and busier urban environments explain why people are getting larger. In Osaka, people can describe in detail the key demands on urban company men to be at work and attend work events that reflect a very competitive economy with highly gendered roles; they can also describe the ways that unhealthy food has proliferated in the cityscape. In Apia and north Georgia, people fully recognize how urbanization and (exclusionary) economic development have driven health-damaging changes in food, exercise, stress, and disconnection from tradition. In Encarnación, the food environment has changed due to dam-related displacement and the resulting growth of the tourist-service economy (including its growing fast food sector). People in all these places, therefore, reflect a high level of awareness of the structural factors that scientists have identified as explaining population-level trends driving excess weight and that define the particularities of weight patterns that emerge in local environments. These are the factors that must be addressed to create widespread weight loss at the population level – if that is the goal.

Yet, despite the seemingly global awareness of these structural factors in driving wider trends toward obesity, the ways in which people engage with the idea of fat in their own lives is framed far more in terms of a model of individual responsibility and blame, even while they express quite complex critiques of historic structural changes. This seems to reflect the ways that Obesity interventions are designed, particularly within biomedicine, as interventions that emphasize that people *themselves* should eat less and exercise more. Clearly, that message has been efficiently transmitted around the world, and people apply it to themselves and others constantly. It is promulgated in the way an Osakan housewife talks to her husband about his weight, and in the way she internalizes his lack of health as her own failing. It is reinforced in the way a Paraguayan soccer player teases his teammate about the size of his belly. Consequently, one of our observations here is that most conversations about weight, even those done with care and concern, overfocus on individuals. In doing so, we argue, they miss the point.

What we see from examining the four case studies through comparison is that this notion of individual responsibility and blame around fat undermines any chance to make real and lasting changes to weight that can actually improve people's health. Some social scientists view the clustering of high Obesity rates in specific locations related to structural inequalities (like low income or racial discrimination) as a signal of environmental or social injustice. A public sense of outrage against governmental infrastructure and policy is muted as over time people have internalized the problem as being of their own doing – their food choices, eating habits, and exercise behaviors. People in our sites talked about their own or others' individual "risky" behaviors. Rather than focusing on a lack of health, some participants across our sites focused on fat, which was entangled with many issues that seemed more pressing than health (such as lack of time, uneven and unpredictable access to nutritious food, or generalized stress).

With this in mind, it is hard to imagine how there can be much political will to address the structural causes of chronic diseases – perhaps most especially in the communities that are the most at risk. If people blame themselves for being fat and then conflate fatness with disease, they are unlikely to take action with the goal of the institutional changes (in medical practice, in government investments) that science suggests are those most likely to positively affect the global population's health. What's needed, obesity experts argue, is improving nationalized health systems, focusing health care on prevention, creating more walkable green spaces, requiring schools to provide healthier school lunches, shortening work hours, building affordable housing nearer to work spaces, and taxing the powerful Big Food/ Big Drink multinationals that produce and market low nutrition foods globally. A focus on self-blame and fat makes it difficult to advance an approach that addresses underlying health issues brought on by unhealthy infrastructure. A focus on individual responsibility for fat is an injustice that marks broader patterns of socioeconomic inequity across multiple levels and for multiple reasons.

Individual-centered blame and a myopic focus on fat = disease doesn't just get in the way of producing much-needed political change. Blaming the problem on individuals also creates anxiety and shame around high body weights. Fear of being fat and attracting the negative reactions of others can create additional and sometimes very distressing worry and self-doubt. More tellingly still, what we see across the four sites we studied is that much of that pain is created and reinforced by those whose good opinions are cherished. Stigma isn't just what is said or done at the doctor's office or the comments one gets in the street. It is what manifests itself in all kinds of interpersonal relationships, including ones characterized by real affection. Consider Masa, who told Cindi that his mom told him that "if he was poked with a pin" he would "explode." Undoubtedly, Masa frequently heard negative comments about his weight from his mother within his home. Masa's mom may have even thought she was offering constructive feedback, to impel him to be healthier and live a better life. The pernicious nature of "helpful feedback" from intimates is partly what makes fat stigma so powerful.

The widespread localization and internalization of blame is also medically concerning. For one, internalized stigma (self-blame) around fat can have direct negative health effects. It discourages people from going out and becoming active, for fear of being judged. It can trigger anxiety-related eating, and cascade into stress responses that have their own negative effects on health such as increasing inflammation and depression. It can also (via both inflammation and depression and independently of these) worsen chronic ailments like diabetes and cardiovascular disease and it can exacerbate psychologically based eating disorders like anorexia.[3] Indeed, it's an interesting point to consider whether many of the diseases that biomedicine currently describes as "weight-related" are actually exacerbated by high body weight or exacerbated by experiences of fat stigma and accompanying psychosocial stress. Moreover, in the context of this research project, we see no evidence that people identified ways in which feeling shame and self-blame (from others or self-directed) helped them move toward health and well-being.

Importantly, our study shows that people have fully embraced the idea that weight and health are almost always entwined. This doesn't actually map onto medical data and scientific evidence. There are many "normal weight" people with very unhealthy metabolic profiles, like high cholesterol and blood pressure. There are also many ostensibly "Obese" people with excellent health markers. However, this idea clearly follows prevailing medical and social thinking that fully embraces the view that fat people are universally and by definition unhealthy.[4] The enduring belief that fat is unhealthy erases the lived experiences of the people who identify as fat and healthy; at the same time it glosses over really interesting scientific findings that don't support this perspective and model of fat as unhealthy. Reliance on biometric measures that define normal levels of blood pressure, cholesterol, and glucose (to list only a few) as healthy based on statistical averages actually contradicts the latest advances in medicine. New personalized and medical interventions are based squarely on the idea of working from an individual's own normal averages, and not on population-based averages. All of this is to say that it is clear that fat itself and fat bodies are negatively valued and that biometric measurements often serve to frame the story in a particular way that suits prevailing medical thinking.

There are, as we noted in the introduction, various forms of activist-driven fat acceptance movements that push back against anti-fat norms. Often these efforts to redefine norms of what is acceptable are based on concerns around weight-related discrimination and, to date, they have been particularly active in countries like the United States, Australia, the United Kingdom, and so on – highly fat stigmatizing Western contexts with widespread social buy-in around certain white norms, in other words. Activists in these places seek to change shared norms and practices around socially acceptable bodies. They recognize that worry about weight is itself medically unhealthy in many contexts (e.g., exacerbating unlikely-to-work crash dieting, or triggering depression). These movements are often spearheaded by people with very large bodies. A core idea is that the moral and medical aspects of weight need to be separated. In north Georgia, some of our participants were aware of this as a movement and felt that the idea of fat being positive and powerful had significantly impacted younger generations and their views of fat. They suggested that fat shaming is lessening, leading to a better situation than that in which they were reared.

There are still other spaces where fat can be viewed as positive and powerful, even if these attitudes, too, are changing.[5] In the Samoa site, large bodies were considered dignified, indicating the generosity and love that a family provided as they cared for an individual over the life course. In the Paraguay site, the association of fat with wealth and privilege was in living memory and was felt still by people struggling with food insecurity and low incomes. Our own previous work in contexts as diverse as South Africa and the United Arab Emirates indicates that people may have absorbed some medicalized ideas about the risks of Obesity and social media/global media–generated ideas about fat being displeasing, but they have not done so uncritically and wholesale: more generous interpretations of large body size, especially in older generations, still linger.

In Japan, people mentioned ways in which those who are *futotteru* could be seen in a positive way if they were cheerful and energetic (*akarukute genki*), but the notion of fat acceptance that wasn't anchored in a known individual was absent from any stated possibility. In other words, knowing someone at the individual level – having a fat friend – can overcome the negative value of the socially stigmatized large body. Indeed, if we consider women comedians in Japan, the most popular and well-known are large-bodied. Perhaps as is to be expected, their (large) bodies are sometimes the punchline. This idea that people we know individually can be valued in spite of their large bodies is undergirded by ideologies of exceptionalism that do not contribute to the larger social level of valuing all members regardless of body size.

The social value placed on body size varies from place to place. For those seeking to build a world that embraces more diversity in its ideas about acceptable and healthy bodies, these findings suggest that Western-style fat-acceptance activism may not be the only way forward. The idea that large bodies can occupy social roles that are highly valued has deep historical roots in many societies and may provide another point of entry into the struggle against fat stigma. This is also suggested by the socially valued roles assigned to people with large bodies – as strong, as caregivers, as part of the social fabric – in places like Samoa. This could create space for a more inclusive form of bodily acceptance.

Finally, we need to return to the basic challenge of understanding how people across the globe conceptualize and respond to weight.

By looking cross culturally at four different sites, in Japan, the United States, Paraguay, and Samoa, we found that worry about weight is pervasive but with social, cultural, political, and economic divides. We found that people are daily juggling multiple dynamics that impact their eating and activity habits. We also found deep understanding of the structural situation by our interviewees across all sites. It is people like those we interviewed who are the experts on their own communities. The grounded understandings that they expressed need to be systematically recognized and then better translated and applied to policy, programmatic, and structural changes.

Appendix A: Five Ethnographers with Five Perspectives

As five anthropologists, we all came to this project having each spent years doing ethnography and interviews in different parts of the world. Bringing five ethnographers together to systematically compare the everyday experiences of fat in four countries is not the standard way most anthropological fieldwork proceeds. It required extra levels of planning and coordination at all phases of the project. Given our distinct training and interests, we each examine fat in slightly different ways. Even working from the same set of interview questions and participant-observation priorities, as we did in this *Fat in Four Cultures* project, we sometimes interpreted the things we saw and heard differently.

Cindi is a linguistic anthropologist who has spent most of her career studying language interaction, gender (specifically masculinity), and Japan.[1] For her, language mediates the social lives of all humans, allowing us to express social relations, status, and identities that include such categories as race, gender, and fatness/obesity. She understands our bodies as one of our central semiotic (meaning-making) systems, expressing just how important language is to the body. For Cindi, giving attention to how people talk about their own and others' bodies sheds light on how they see themselves vis-à-vis the others in their local and global communities. Some of Cindi's work has examined the ways in which people use Japanese language forms to indicate particular kinds of identities (e.g., regional or gendered identities).

When Cindi turned her attention to language and fat within the context of Japan, she became particularly interested in the ways that people narrate what it means to be large or small.[2] For example, consider the difference between claiming to be chubby rather than fat. In Japan, people drew a strong distinction between these two terms, allowing chubby (*pocchari*) a slightly more positive valence on the body size continuum while fat (*futotteru*) clearly held a negative valence. Paying attention to the ways in which people use language (including silence) highlights the ways in which they demarcate their particular identities across time and space.

Alex is trained in both biological and cultural anthropology and thinks at the intersection of the two, examining how culture shapes human biology – a field called biocultural anthropology. For example, her recent work focusing on weight-related stigma considered the ways in which particular physical traits are read and interpreted in specific sociocultural contexts as unacceptable and immoral, and ultimately how these cultural meanings act to shape health outcomes like depression or chronic disease.[3] She has worked in multiple sites in Oceania and in the United States and in many other countries over the last three decades,[4] and much of her ethnographic work included direct measurement of body size and considered its health implications. Alex thus has the most diverse ethnographic portfolio of the five of us and has been working on issues around weight the longest; she is particularly interested in and attuned to detecting broader cultural patterns. She is also the most versed of us all in thinking about Obesity in clinical terms and has the most experience and comfort connecting to medical and public health experts and the ways they view patients' bodies.[5]

Jessica studies the social life of health. While medical approaches to health tend to focus on the metrics of the body as indicators of health or disease, Jessica looks at how people understand the ways that social and economic contexts shape the distribution of disease and develop critiques of their worlds as a result. This means she explores the manifold ways that people create health through their caring relations in ways that, contrary to appearances, don't always seem like they are about health in the biomedical sense.[6] In other words, she looks at how health, as an idea, is constructed and practiced across diverse contexts from clinics to churches, and from hospitals to households. In Samoa, this has led her to study the intersection of faith and medicine, exploring how Christian practice shapes experiences of well-being.[7] She has examined how churches play a central role in sustaining, and sometimes constraining, health. As a critical medical anthropologist, this means considering how unequal access to life chances, in terms of food and medicine and social support, is part of how people make meaning of the lived experiences of their bodies. As such, an additional focus of her work is on the culture and consequences of health promotion, in particular the ways that public health messaging creates normative ways of thinking about health, especially weight and body size.[8]

Sarah's past fieldwork has examined college students' attitudes to and conversations around weight and fat in the United Arab Emirates[9] and the United States.[10] She also spent several years exploring the experiences of individuals undergoing bariatric surgery, following prospective patients through their gastric bypasses and subsequent weight loss, and analyzing their shifting experiences of stigma and health.[11] Of all of us, she has the most ethnographic experience with people living with extreme body weight. This fits with her focus on the ways that suffering and inequality intersect with health and resiliency in people's everyday lives. Weight, chronic disease, and fatness are interesting points of entry to examine these sometimes contradictory, sometimes complementary, forces because at this particular point in time their health implications are inextricably bound up with assumptions about morality, personal and familial worth, and responsibility. For example, popular media in the United States right now contains all kinds of pain-filled accounts of what it means to be fat – and the daily experiences of fat-based discrimination and stigma intertwine with concerns that are framed as more explicitly medical (such as diabetes). Sarah accordingly has also led our team studies on how weight and culture intersect in virtual online communities.[12]

Amber is an anthropologist with expertise in economic, ecological, and medical anthropology. Her work is broadly concerned with how people get the resources they need to survive, and what happens when people can't get what they need for a safe, healthy, and productive life. Much of her work has focused on people's essential needs for food and water. She has examined how water and food access are embedded in cultural and social systems and often uses cross-cultural research designs.[13] For example, she has examined how people who have no water pipes get water "off the grid," how people use sharing relationships to get food, and how being water- and food-insecure harms people's mental health and well-being.[14] While collaborating with Alex on a study among Latinx immigrants in the United States a decade ago (conducting a kind of research called community-based participatory research), Amber was surprised that people explained food insecurity and obesity as distressing twin threats: for those interviewed, being poor meant buying cheap food, and cheap food meant getting fat and sick. Since then, Amber has studied how and why poverty and fatness together act to impede people's access to health, wealth, and dignity. As an anthropological methodologist, Amber has developed new approaches to sampling, collecting, and analyzing cross-cultural data within the field, some of which we used in the research that informs this book.

What we each see as anthropologists is, of course, not just about our different theoretical orientations. It is also shaped by our own personal histories, values, and physical bodies. It means that even when we used exactly the same set of interview questions and theoretical approach within our four field sites to study fatness, each of us highlighted slightly different complexities and contradictions that were pivotal to understanding whether, and how, fat mattered in people's lives in a particular place.

Appendix B: Research Methods

In bringing together a team of ethnographers, we tried to push forward the systematic aspects of research, focusing on developing a shared sampling and interview protocol that built on local ethnographic knowledge. Studies that use secondary (i.e., already collected) data to devise across-site comparisons are often hobbled by lack of context[15] and an inability to directly compare disparate forms of evidence. We worked purposefully and diligently to solve the triple problems of ensuring that comparative data had context, designing a protocol that was ethnographically informed, and ensuring that comparisons were not misinterpreted. Table B.1 provides the full suite of the methods we deployed at each site and in the post-fieldwork analysis, and why we selected them.

By focusing on the purposeful collection of data that relied on a protocol that had been thoughtfully and collaboratively developed over many conversations and well-tested before we went to the field, we were able to avoid some potential pitfalls of cross-cultural comparative ethnography. These pitfalls include decontextualization, which refers to the process of removing data from their context in ways that compromise the validity of the findings. This is especially problematic for ethnographic data because contextual information is so important for analysis and interpretation.

Decontextualization, mistranslation, and other analytic errors can lead to another possible pitfall of comparative scholarship:

Table B.1. Research activities and their justifications

What we did	Why we did it
Participant-observation	Learn from living, being with, and observing people
Write field notes	Capture data collected from participant-observation, in narrative text, photos, drawings, and early theme analysis
Develop interview protocol	Through team discussions, discover possible similarities and differences and construct a protocol for systematic semi-structured interviewing across field sites
Pilot interview protocol	Determine if the interview protocol is understandable to participants and elicits data in the ways we envisioned; revise the protocol until it works for us and for participants
Translate and back-translate interview protocol	Translate the interview protocol from English to the field language (and/or language variety); have a second fluent speaker of the field language translate back to English to ensure translations are understandable, accurate, and complete
Purposive sample	Compose a purposive (nonrandom) sample that allows us to compare interview themes across sites and interview responses within sites (here, across age and gender)
Semi-structured interviews	Collect data on participants' views and experiences with open-ended response formats, using a semi-structured protocol that facilitates comparisons within and across sites
Data recording and transcription	Capture conversations that occur during semi-structured interviews and convert them into textual transcripts that can be more easily analyzed in qualitative analysis software
Theme identification	Using participant-observation and interview data, identify important meanings within each field site
Meta-thematic analysis	Comparative theme analysis to identify meta-themes (or themes shared across field sites) and site-specific themes
Cross-cultural comparison	Comparative ethnographic analysis to understand and contextualize similarities/differences in topics across sites
Thick description	Descriptive analysis and writing that helps the reader understand and contextualize participant-observation data
Ethnographic vignettes	Brief story or description of an event from the participant-observation that illuminates important cross-cutting themes or findings from the analysis
Ethnographic interpretation and theoretical integration	Through iterative team discussions, explore and clarify convergences around the four core domains
Data translation	Translate the data from the original field language to English; this is a final step used to render the interview data, ethnographic vignettes, and thick description understandable to an English-language reader

misinterpretation. When data are translated and coded for analysis, the chances of misinterpreting the data can increase, especially if these steps are not performed rigorously. Because each of us had long-standing experience in each of our field sites, we were able to keep the primary data more closely situated within their context while doing analysis. There was also overlap in expertise across some of the sites, which was incredibly helpful. Alex has previously worked in the Pacific, including Samoa, in Latin America, and in Georgia; and during this research on fat, she also visited Japan with Cindi. This overlap was important to how the dynamic of comparing and integrating the study sites evolved, and helped us mitigate misinterpretation. Moreover, because we worked as a team to build the analytic framework, we were able to take advantage of non-site-specific experts to contribute to analysis without decontextualizing the data (i.e., those who didn't know the other sites). To us, the long-term knowledge across the sites was key to the interpretation, but the comparable semi-structured qualitative data were necessary to create a rigorous cross-cultural analysis.

HOW WE COLLECTED THE DATA

To kick off the data collection, Sarah went to north Georgia for two weeks, to recruit participants and to pilot the interview protocols. Recruitment and interviews went smoothly and after reviewing the data together, the team decided to roll out data collection across all the sites. Sarah subsequently went to Georgia twice more over the course of eighteen months (each trip lasting about eight days), once by herself and once with Alex. Alex, who has over twenty years of ethnographic experience in Georgia, went with Sarah on the second trip, to help with recruitment, to flesh out participant-observation there, and to visit her family. Together, the two of them recruited and interviewed twenty-two people (eighteen women and four men) for this project, spread across the peri-urban arc of northern Georgia above Atlanta. Once we had all done an early review of the Georgia data and discussed lessons learned, Cindi, Jessica, and Amber spent the summer of 2017 in their respective field sites, each interviewing a minimum of sixteen people (twelve women, four men) using the same interview protocol.

DEVELOPING THE INTERVIEW PROTOCOL

We began our collaboration with some very practical, earned understandings of what people are generally willing and able to share about their bodies. Drawing on this knowledge, we worked together to select domains of knowledge that we agreed people across our diverse field sites would understand, recognize, and be willing to share. Based on our own prior fieldwork experiences, plus a detailed understanding of the international anthropological literature on weight, fat, and obesity, we identified four key domains around which the interviews were organized. By domains, we mean thematic areas of concern. The four domains – (1) food and eating, (2) body ideals and body capital, (3) disease and health, (4) stigma and fat talk – helped us organize and clarify the shared categories of the interviews across the sites. The domains were also selected for their theoretical relevance, meaning they explored areas that anthropologists working in an array of places globally have identified previously as salient for how bodies matter most in peoples' lives. Having an organized, semi-structured protocol also ensured that once data were collected and ready for analysis, we could engage in rigorous and commensurate cross-cultural comparisons.

SEMI-STRUCTURED INTERVIEWS

In ethnographic interviews, a goal is to elicit as much data as possible to describe people's shared (cultural) and personal understandings of the world, and in their own words. In this study, we purposefully used semi-structured interviews, where each participant is asked to respond in the same order to the same set of questions. Using a semi-structured interview guide combined the advantages of open-ended ethnographic interviewing – that lets people take the lead on where the conversation is going – with the comparability gained from having structured responses from participants and thus more directly comparable material from each site to analyze.

The interview questions were designed to get people across the sites thinking and talking about the topics presented, encouraging them to discuss the topics in as much detail as possible. A carefully curated set of open-ended questions began that process (see appendix C). Much ethnography can be done off-the-cuff, using unstructured interview techniques that follow the participants' leads. But our case required different techniques. In comparative work, it is imperative that the interviews yield reliable, comparable qualitative data in an analyzable format. For us, this meant using a semi-structured interview guide. But, we all also followed new leads as they came up in interviews, asking for more detail on interesting or unexpected revelations. It was up to each of us as researchers to use techniques to get the person to talk in more detail and with more depth. This included verbal probes like "Why do you say that?" "Can you tell me more?" or "Has it always been like that?" But, in Samoa, for example, an eyebrow raise is a key probe technique – it shows you are listening, value what is being said, and want people to continue. Active listening is fundamental; this includes giving feedback through nodding, smiling, or other listening cues to encourage participants to keep thinking out loud. We recorded everything the participants said. Once transcribed, the detailed transcripts of what people said become the basis on which systematic analysis could be conducted.

PARTICIPANT-OBSERVATION

Another tool that allows us to better understand and contextualize the interview data is long-term participant-observation. Participant-observation is a method in which the researcher learns about a community and the people in it by doing things with participants, living everyday life, and recording her observations using field notes. When Cindi was in Japan, for example, she wasn't simply interviewing people with the set of questions. She met friends in the train station for *yakitori* (grilled chicken on skewers), visited colleagues at Japanese universities, paid utility bills at the nearby *konbini* (convenience store), and interacted with friends on Japanese social media. In all these contexts, Cindi had additional opportunities to gain critical insights into basic norms and rules of everyday Japanese life. These activities, therefore, are all part of participant-observation, a hallmark of ethnography in particular, and qualitative research methods in general.

Participant-observation relies on researchers embedding themselves into the community from which interview participants will ultimately come. It allows us as researchers to gain familiarity with the particular values, routines, and common-sense understandings of the people in the community. It also requires language and cultural competence, and *participation* (not just observation at a distance, as one might do in a lab) from a researcher. In doing so, we are forced to reiteratively refine our competencies over time and space as we come and go from our field sites. In short, participant-observation allows us to go about our daily lives as if we were part of the local community while simultaneously keeping an awareness of ourselves that we are not part of the community. Participant observation provides a constant source of internal interrogation and self-reflection. It also teaches us to see, hear, and observe behaviors and to systematically document these in our field notes (discussed below). For example, participants in Paraguay often told Amber that they tried to feed their children a nutritious and balanced diet. Amber, however, while socializing in the community, observed parents giving their children foods they had specifically labeled as sweets and junk food, like candy, potato chips, and soda pop (at the same time that Amber was allowing her own children to also eat these foods). Participant-observation is critical to the analysis of the data in that it can provide context for behaviors that are claimed or asserted by participants in a formal interview setting but are contradicted by daily observations.

INTERVIEW SAMPLE

The purpose of sampling is to make sure that the data sources (in this case, interviews) are selected so that we can make credible conclusions.[16] In our work for this project, we were interested in describing cultural norms around food and fat, in terms of how they varied within and across cultures.

Our study uses a purposive sample, meaning each of us selected our interviewees based on pre-specified targets of gender and age. We expected gender and age would be among the most important criteria for predicting disparate views around fat and would be relevant to participants in all four sites. Some factors are crucially important for understanding cultural views on fat in one society but are largely meaningless in other societies. For example, race is a very important social category within the United States, perhaps especially in the American South, where we did fieldwork. But it isn't an important social category in Paraguay, and racial categories in Japan are mostly just used to distinguish those who are Japanese from non-Japanese foreigners. In other words, "race" wasn't a good way to compare interviewees' views on fat across our field sites because race meant such different things to the locals in each place.

In each site, we interviewed a minimum of twelve women: at least six women under forty-five years old (roughly, younger than middle age) and at least six women forty-five years old and over (roughly, middle aged and older) (see table B.2). We chose this number because research shows that between six and twelve interview participants are needed to conduct thematic analysis.[17] Within each age bracket, we selected each woman based on her ability to provide new insights into the ways that socioeconomic status intersects with cultural views on food and fat. For example, Amber started by interviewing three food-secure, middle-class women who were under forty-five. After that, she added two women who were food-insecure and one very wealthy woman to round out the under-forty-five sample. In addition to the women, we also interviewed at least four men in each site: two spouses of women over forty-five years old and two spouses of women under forty-five years old. These men were included to get a male perspective on the phenomena discussed in their wives' interviews.

This sample design is ideal for comparing views across age classes within each site, and to some extent gender and socioeconomic status. One drawback to this sampling design is that it limits our ability to describe variability in many important ways. We do not have enough variability to describe men's views distinctly, but only in relation to those of the women. We have only one unmarried man in the sample (from Osaka, Japan). We also have no same-sex couples or gender-nonconforming participants. In addition, our research design does not support structured comparisons on potentially important factors that were not explicit selection criteria (e.g., not just race, but religion, parenthood, living arrangements, sexuality, etc.).

Table B.2. Participant descriptions, minimum *N*, sampling, ages*

Age	Women	Men
Young (44 and below)	6	2 (these are coupled with 2 of the 6 women)
Middle-aged and older (45 and older)	6	2 (these are coupled with 2 of the 6 women)

Total *N* for interviews per site = 16 (12 women, 4 men; 4 couples).
Total *N* for interviews = 64 (48 women, 16 men; 16 couples).
Inclusion for participation across each site: long-term residence in site; long exposure to site norms; socialized to the area and the norms.
*A full description of all participants across all sites is provided in appendix D.

DATA MANAGEMENT: FIELD NOTES, INTERVIEWS, TRANSCRIPTIONS, AND TRANSLATIONS

Writing Field Notes

Field notes documented what happened at each field site during the fieldwork season. These provided an additional dataset that helped describe, interpret, and explain what emerged in the interviews. Each researcher had her own system for producing field notes. Outside the interviews, Cindi took handwritten field notes over the course of each day throughout her movements. For this project, while out and about in Japan (riding trains, sitting in cafés, walking to and from interview locations), Cindi paid particular attention to body size, built infrastructure, and especially how the people around her were reacting to these aspects of daily life. Did she observe and/or overhear Japanese people staring or remarking on the body sizes of the other people moving about the various contexts? What kinds of remarks or behavior did people exhibit around non-normatively small or large bodies? How did children behave in public around non-normatively sized bodies? How might remarks and behaviors shift depending on the gender/sex of the non-normative body? These kinds of observations made up quite a bit of the field notes collected when not doing interviews. Cindi also took field notes during the interviews. At the start of each interview, Cindi recorded where the interview was taking place, who she was talking to, and any specialized terms that the participant used during the course of the interview. Finally, at the end of each day, Cindi wrote up summaries of her notes; these were done on a computer with reference to the handwritten notes.

Jessica similarly took handwritten notes during the day and during interviews; these were keywords and other memory aids for later description. At the end of each day, she then created a log of interactions, people, and places, with longer descriptions of the observations that were keyworded in the handwritten notes. During each of Sarah's three trips to the US site in Georgia, she too typed up daily field notes on her laptop, fleshing them out with photos (omitting identifiable people) she took throughout the day with her iPhone. On the first and third trip, when Sarah was staying at the house of a local friend, she would ask the friend to comment on the field notes (which meant that the notes necessarily contained no confidential information from the audio-recorded interviews). On the second trip to Georgia, Alex and Sarah went together. Sarah again typed up daily field notes, and asked Alex (who was related to and/or knew many of the individuals, families, and communities in the fieldwork area) for clarification and expansion on many emerging themes. Additionally, Alex kept running notes on what she heard and saw during her visit. She also added annotated comments based on her years of experience in the field. She then created one massive set of field notes at the end of that second trip, which she sent to Sarah. The result: a dense set of field notes triangulating multiple viewpoints.

Amber used voice recognition software on her smartphone to auto-dictate data collected from participant-observation and to transcribe (while still in the field) conversations she had just heard. The smartphone also enabled her to capture photos and directly upload them to qualitative analysis software immediately. Before, during, and after interviews, Amber used field notes to record key observations that could not be captured by the transcript. She also kept a running document with emerging themes she uncovered during participant-observation and interviews.

As this shows, field notes are a somewhat idiosyncratic and personal form of data collection, and may not be an ideal form of data for direct comparison across field sites. However, they are still essential to this analysis because they enabled us to capture observed settings, behavior, and conversations and they provide context for the self-reported data, where people inevitably try to present themselves in the best light (wouldn't you?). In addition, the field notes enabled us to "write thick description" (an anthropological stock phrase that refers to our ability to provide a richly described and analyzed moment in time) and develop ethnographic vignettes that are important for sharing the field site with our readers.

Recording Interview Data

The interviews themselves were recorded using iPod recorders, with attached external microphones as needed. We chose Apple technology for this project for two reasons: (1) In the past, some of us have had problems with proprietary digital data formats that went out of date and became inaccessible. We reasoned that the Apple file formats might have a longer digital life, when compared to other recording choices. (2) Apple products like the iPhone are now globally recognized and familiar; as such, audio recording with an Apple device meant that each participant was familiar with such a device sitting on a table. People did not pay close attention to the device and were not bothered by it. Each researcher immediately backed up her files after finishing an interview. We did not, however, back them up to our personal iCloud storage. We mention this because it's an important thing for researchers to keep in mind in an age of casual and constant informational exchange and backups. After completion of all interviews, the files (with the real names of the interviewees removed) were sent to ASU Obesity Solutions, where a coordinator centrally managed and backed up the files. Then, all files were sent to external services for transcription.

Transcription

We used external transcription services to produce transcripts of the interview data. Transcription can be an important analytic moment in qualitative research, so it is worth explaining why we chose this approach (rather than transcribing the interviews ourselves). Each researcher took field notes and/or did theme identification during or immediately after her interviews. As a result, all of the interviews had already been initially analyzed before the transcription began (making another round of pre-analysis largely redundant). Another advantage of using an external service is that transcription style is the same across all four field sites. In our case, transcripts captured the interviews verbatim (e.g., with pauses, laughter, production errors) as this was the level of detail appropriate to our analysis plan.

However, as is true of all recorded interviews and their transcripts, they do not actually reproduce the moment-to-moment interaction of the interview. Transcripts are also decontextualized, in the sense that the words people said are removed from socially meaningful information about who said them where, how they were said, and what nonverbal gestures and meanings were communicated. All of us used field notes to fill in some of the data loss and capture key observations of nonverbal data. That said, *all* data are decontextualized, as the purpose of collecting data is to distill the complexities of day-to-day life to a more concise and analyzable record.

Finally, when we do our own transcription, we generally build in a system of cross-checks in which a secondary analyst ensures that the initial transcript is accurate. In this case, we did not have in-house researchers available to do cross-checks of our research languages and varieties (e.g., Osakan Japanese; Paraguayan Spanish; Samoan). For these reasons, we determined high-quality external transcription services would be appropriate for our cross-cultural interview data, allowing us to become the cross-check on completion of the transcript.

Data Translation

Translation (in this case, changing non-English transcripts into English) can be a problem because it decontextualizes the data, increasing the distance of the data from their original source and losing some of the original meaning in the conversations. For example, when someone talks in Japanese about the *depāto no resutoran gai*, we can translate this into English as "the restaurant floor of the department store." However, the English translation loses a lot of the original meaning, which is intimately connected to the reality of a department store in Japan (usually an eight or nine story building with lavish displays of goods), which always has a restaurant floor or floors near the top of the building. These restaurant floors contain multiple individual eating establishments offering an array of cuisines from Italian, French, or Spanish, to Chinese, Korean, or Japanese. Department stores in Japan are very different spaces than they are in the United States; they are points of destination not just for shopping but for lavish consumption of food and drink. These meanings are, of course, implicitly understood by Japanese people (or others familiar with Japan), but cannot be quickly conveyed in English.

For this reason, all data were initially analyzed in the original interview language: Japanese in Japan, Spanish with Jopara (a combination of the indigenous language Guarani and Spanish) in Paraguay, mostly English with some Samoan in Samoa, and English in the United States. We kept the data in the original interview language through many analytic phases, including theme analysis and write-up. Once we had final drafts of our written chapters, we translated direct quotes from the original interview language to English. We used our own socially located English varieties in these translations, rather than trying to imitate or convert the interviewees' language varieties to parallel social locations that exist in English. Amber, Cindi, and Jessica cross-checked their translations with native speakers of their field site languages (Spanish/Jopara, Japanese, and Samoan, respectively).

DATA ANALYSIS

Fieldwork was done alone or in teams of two. The process of data analysis was fully collaborative. Over the course of one year, we gathered together three times to workshop for several days to analyze and interpret the larger dataset we had compiled from the four sites.

THEME IDENTIFICATION

Using data from participant-observation and semi-structured interviews, we each began with individual processes of theme identification. Identifying themes is about finding the underlying shared meanings that cut across many experiences or narratives. In our case, like many anthropologists studying their field data, we used many different techniques to identify themes.[18] The first, and most common approach, was to look for common or repeated motifs. For example, the idea that one's own weight is an individual responsibility is a theme that was repeated in each of our field sites. Another technique we often used was to look for concepts shared across cultural in-groups. For example, Amber found the concept of *buena presencia* in Spanish (which translates literally to "good presence") to be a euphemism often used in job interviews to indicate that only thin, good-looking people would get the job. This suggests a theme around job discrimination and the economic value of thin bodies. We also looked for metaphors and similes that people used in their interviews and in day-to-day life. For example, Cindi was told that thin people look *gari-gari*, which is a mimetic expression meaning "like a skeleton." This suggests a theme that a very thin body is not ideal but rather is frightening. After each of us completed this phase of analysis, we each compiled a list of around thirty descriptive themes describing key meanings around food and fat that emerged as most relevant in our own field site.

META-THEMATIC ANALYSIS

After individually identifying themes for our field sites, we then collated and integrated them. Each theme was printed on an index card, which resulted in five sets of pile sort index cards (one from each ethnographer).[19] Meta-themes are cross-cutting meanings around fat that could be found in all sites. We began first by doing a pile sort activity in which each researcher separately and individually sorted the index cards from all four field sites into piles that contained cross-cutting meanings. For example, one such emergent pile dealt with anguish over children's eating and bodies. After we had all completed our sorting, we presented our piles to each other and explained how and why we composed each pile. This produced a dynamic conversation in which we debated, argued, and came to consensus around the major themes emerging from our participant-observation and semi-structured interview data across all four field sites.

CROSS-CULTURAL COMPARISONS

As part of our conversations about meta-themes, we also were implicitly conducting many cross-cultural comparisons. We had to talk through how and why things were different among the field sites. This phase of our research produced many surprises and important epiphanies, where we (as lead ethnographers who had worked for many years in our field sites) were challenged to see food, fat, and our sites in new ways. For example, Cindi observed that people in her Japanese field site expressed concern for people with large bodies, often saying *ano hito wa genki ka dō ka*, "I just wonder if that person is healthy or not." Sarah then questioned this, saying that this may not really be an expression of concern; rather, it is a form of shaming people with large bodies. Amber then noticed that people in her Paraguayan field site also expressed this concern in this way and wondered if it might also carry a hidden meaning of shaming or stigma. One advantage we had was some overlap in site expertise. For example, Alex and Jessica both have a lot of experience working in the Pacific Islands, including Samoa, and Sarah and Alex had both done research in Georgia. Our analysis thus came out of a long process of interrogating each assumption we made about what we observed in the field.

Appendix C: *Fat in Four Cultures* Interview Protocol

We include this protocol because ethnographic research is often a black box, so to speak. In other words, the history of anthropology rooted in an individual, lone ethnographer model often obscures the actual day-to-day work of fieldwork. We include our protocol to enhance scientific transparency and to provide students with a model.

PROTOCOL BEGIN

Tell me about yourself:
- How old are you?
- Where were you born? Where do you live now?
- What level of education have you completed?
- What kind of work do you do?

Tell me about your family:
- Are you married?
- Do you have children?
- Who do you live with?

Protocol domains and questions:
    I'd like to ask you some questions about food.

1. Food and Eating

Q1: Do you think the kinds of foods people eat around here have changed over time? Could you tell me about some "traditional foods" that used to be consumed frequently but now are not?

Q2: In the past in (SITE), what did a typical breakfast look like? Lunch? Supper/Dinner?

Q3: What about now? Could you take me through what a typical day of "eating" looks like for you? A typical meal (breakfast, lunch, dinner)?

Q4: Do you think the way you eat is typical of people your age who live around here? Why/Why not?

Q5: Does this type of eating match what you think you should be eating? Does how you currently eat match what you would like to eat? Follow up: Why is there a difference between what you think you should eat and what you *do* eat?

Q6: Who does most of the grocery shopping in your family? Who does most of the cooking? Who makes decisions about what you eat? Do you feel these are good choices?

Prompts:

PARAGUAY: Change since the 1980s [end of the Strossner dictatorship]?

RURAL GA: Would you say you eat mainly a traditional Southern diet (how, when, what, when not)? How important is it to you that you get to be able to eat traditional Southern foods? Why?

JPN: Western vs. Japanese diet? What about *wagashi* (Japanese sweets) vs. *yogashi* (Western sweets)?

Transition question: Do the foods people eat affect their bodies? How? Which foods? Are some foods healthier than others? Is the effect different today than it was in the past? [Getting at rule-based ideas.]

2. Body Ideals/Body Capital

Q1: What kinds of bodies do you think Samoans/Japanese/Americans and Southerners/Paraguayans in general most want to have? Why?

Q2: What does the ideal male/female (masculine/feminine) body look like? Have ideas about beauty and ideal bodies changed over time in America? Georgia? How? What about particular body parts?

Q3: Are there particular jobs or situations where it is better to be smaller or bigger? Work/making an income; women; men; older/younger women/men? Or, give an example from researcher's context to try to make analogy for participant.

Prompts:

PARAGUAY: Could it hurt people's incomes if they don't look this way? [Prompt: urban vs. rural]

JPN: Traditional body ideals vs. contemporary ideals; rural vs. urban.

Now I'd like to ask you a bit about your health.

3. Disease/Health of Large Bodies

Q1: Do you consider yourself healthy? Why/why not?

Q2: Has a doctor (or nurse, etc.) ever suggested that you should reduce your body size (lose weight)? Can you tell me about that?

Q3: Have you ever been diagnosed with any disease that you think is related to your weight? Can you tell me about that?

Q4: What diseases do you think are related to weight? Are men/women more likely to get them? Are Samoans/Japanese/Americans and Southerners/Paraguayans more likely to get these diseases than other groups of people? Why?

Q5: Do you think you yourself or people in your family are at risk of any of these diseases? Why?

Q6: Are there times when being fat can be healthy? For example, is being fat healthy when you are young? Do you think being fat is healthier for men/women?

PARAGUAY: Has the diabetes situation changed much since the 1980s?

RURAL GA: How would you feel if a doctor told you that you needed to lose weight?

JPN: Do you think women are usually healthier than men? Why (alcohol consumption)? Gout?

SAMOA: Why do people get NCDs (non-communicable diseases)?

Now I am going to ask some questions about bodies in general in SITE society.

4. Bodies, Self, and Society

Q1: Are there some sizes of bodies that are disadvantaged in SITE society? (Prompt: Are there particular kinds of bodies that get made fun of? Are some types of bodies treated differently by people (such as in the schoolyard or workplace)?

Q2: What do you think of your friends who have thin/large bodies? Your family? Strangers? Have you ever heard people complain about thin/large bodies?

Q3: How do you feel being around other people with thin/large bodies? Does it make you feel comfortable? Uncomfortable? Do you ever avoid people with thin/large bodies?

Q4: When you see a stranger in public that is very thin/large, what is the first thought that runs through your mind? Do you ever feel like there aré places people with thin/large bodies shouldn't go?

Q5: If someone is overweight (or underweight?), whose responsibility is it? Follow up: Do you think it is important for society to be concerned about people's weight?

PARAGUAY: What kind of body would you be proud for your [spouse] or [son/daughter] to have? Would it be embarrassing for them to have a body that is bigger than [the one described]? Why – how – can you think of an example?

RURAL GA: What if you ran into a friend who had gained a lot of weight since you last saw them?

JPN: Sitting on the train; at the public bath.

SAMOA: Where do you hear disparaging or positive statements about fat? What kinds of things do you think other people associate with weight?

Now I'd like to talk about how some of these ideas connect to you:

5. General Own-Body Concerns

Q1: Do you ever notice other people's body shapes/sizes? When do you notice other people's body shapes?

Q2: Do you ever notice your own body shape or size? Can you tell me a time when you felt good about/proud of your body? How about a time when you remember not feeling good about your body? Like, do you remember ever feeling embarrassed by your body size or shape?

Q3: Does your body cause you any anxiety or embarrassment when you are around other people? What about when you are alone? Follow-up: Are there spaces where you feel more comfortable about/ in your body than others? Less comfortable?

Q4: Are you happy with your body – how and why? Has any of your family or friends ever suggested that you should reduce your body size (lose weight)? Can you tell me about that?

Q5: Can you think of times when someone else, like a stranger or acquaintance, has commented on your body size? How did you feel? [Prompt: Have you ever felt you were treated differently (better or worse) due to your body size?]

Q6: Do you think this would be different if you were younger/older, male/female, pre/post-reproductive?

Q7: Are there times when you have been proud or felt good about being big? Can you tell me about those?

Q8: If you could change your body in any way, what would you want to change? And how would you like that to be done (e.g., surgery, exercise, diet)? [What is stopping you? etc.]

PARAGUAY: Reproduction vs. agriculture [agricultural labor]. What do bodies that can do these jobs well look like?

RURAL GA: Do you dress for your body? When do you make the most effort to do this?
Follow-up:
Who do you complain to?
Do any of your friends or family complain to you about these kinds of issues?
Do you worry that you are too small/big for xyz activities?
What kind of sports did you enjoy in high school? Do you still occasionally play/engage in that sport?

Finally, I'd like to ask you about who you talk about weight with.

6. Fat Talk (if questions seem too direct, please go directly to prompts listed below)

Q1: Do you ever talk to family members about your body weight or how your body looks? Do they talk to you? Tell me about these conversations. Are they different from the way conversations go with your friends?

Q2: How do you think girls talk about weight and body vs. boys?

Q3: Do you think people who are older/younger than you talk about their weight differently? Do you ever have conversations with people about weight who are not your age?

Potential fat talk prompts depending on situation:

- Does your daughter/son (sister/brother, wife/partner if appropriate) ever ask you if s/he looks fat? How do you respond?
- If you see a good friend who has recently gained/lost a noticeable amount of weight, what do you say about the weight gain/loss?
- Do you complain that your pants are too tight?
- Do you complain about hair loss?

So now I'd like to ask a little bit about your body ...

- How much do you think you weigh? Has that changed over time? When was the last time you were weighed?
- How tall do you think you are?
- Would you classify yourself as underweight/about right/somewhat overweight/extremely overweight? or,
- How would you classify yourself in terms of weight? What about body shape?

PROTOCOL END

Appendix D: Participant Information across All Sites

Site	Woman/Man	Pseudonym	Age	Occupation
Osaka, Japan	Woman	Kikue	63	Professional house cleaning (part-time)
	Woman	Kaori	62	NPO volunteer coordinator
	Woman	Chie	61	Housewife
	Woman	Aya	42	Day-care worker
	Woman	Sachiko	38	Bakery/café worker
	Woman	Kaori	62	Non-profit coordinator (unpaid)
	Woman	Tomoko	27	Freelance graphic design artist
	Woman	Setsuko	31	Office worker
	Woman	Megumi	49	Family business
	Woman	Hitomi	31	Office worker
	Woman	Fumie	23	Health-care industry sales
	Woman	Hikari	32	Elder day-care worker
	Man	Masa	50	Hotel front desk
	Man	Tōru	69	Retired/part-time parking attendant
	Man	Kentaro	65	Retired from hotel management/university professor
	Man	Koichi	40	Insurance company
EXTRA	Man	Daisuke	23	Graduate student
North Georgia, USA	Woman	Caroline	50	Taxi driver
	Woman	Allison	55	Retired from corporate job
	Man	Kevin	61	Retired attorney
	Woman	Christina	20	University student
	Woman	Colleen	20	University student

Site	Woman/Man	Pseudonym	Age	Occupation
	Woman	Donna	62	Administrative office worker
	Woman	Jennifer	50	Health-care laboratory technician
	Woman	Charlene	38	Administrative office worker
	Man	Robert	38	Administrative office worker
	Woman	Rosemary	66	Retired administrative office worker
	Woman	Lily Rose	58	Administrative office worker
	Man	Patrick	72	Retired attorney
	Woman	Anna	25	Administrative office worker
	Man	Paul	25	Retail worker
	Woman	Jean	48	Full-time mother
	Woman	Eleanor	68	Retired teacher
	Woman	Lisa	41	Administrative worker
	Woman	Victoria	21	University student
	Woman	Jennifer	29	University student and full-time mother
	Woman	Leslie	21	University student
	Woman	Kristen	20	University student
	Woman	Amy	28	Administrative office worker
Encarnación, Paraguay	Man	Juan	49	Tailor
	Woman	Denise	35	Cardiology office secretary
	Woman	Antonia	52	Part-time cleaner and housewife
	Woman	Rosa	60	Retired school principal
	Man	Jorge	51	Security guard
	Woman	Estefanía	29	Works in mother's fast food business
	Man	Sergei	44	Mechanic/small business owner
	Woman	Neider	37	Clerk in clothing shop
	Woman	Mia	35	Former owner of plus-size boutique/current college student
	Woman	Zulma	47	Owner of a small laundry
	Woman	Mercedes	31	Former teacher/now stay-at-home mom
	Woman	Elisa	49	Runs clothing business
	Woman	Sofia	58	Housewife/helps in husband's office
	Woman	Maima	20	Housewife
	Woman	Luján	28	Businesswoman (owns multiple large businesses)
	Man	Pacha	33	Businessman (owns multiple large businesses)
EXTRA	Man	Ferdinando	35	Retired soccer player
EXTRA	Man	N/A	33	Nutritionist

Site	Woman/Man	Pseudonym	Age	Occupation
Apia, Samoa	Woman	Katerina	23	Government ministry employee
	Woman	Sina	29	University instructor
	Woman	Alofa	42	University instructor
	Woman	Kilisi	42	Translator/cultural instructor
	Woman	Lanuola	27	Government ministry employee
	Woman	Maria	39	University instructor
	Woman	Princess	36	NGO employee
	Woman	Lusi	35	Government ministry employee
	Woman	Pua	51	Gym owner
	Woman	Malia	61	Caretaker for her husband
	Woman	Tofi	58	Retired university administrator
	Woman	Tausa	66	Retired government ministry executive
	Woman	Lili	68	University administrator
	Woman	Eseta	46	Government ministry executive
	Man	Loto	48	Church ministry staff
	Man	Amosa	38	Fitness instructor/personal trainer
	Man	Peter	72	Agricultural research scientist
	Man	Iona	70	Farmer/household caretaker

Appendix E: Recommendations and Insights

Recommendations for student readers:

- The emotional damage done by the label of fat, such as in undermining the sense that one has value to others, is mostly communicated in social relationships. This includes the nuclear family. Be aware of this and don't fat-shame, even "constructively," and particularly avoid doing this to your children because it can track them for life.
- Talking about bodies opens up the space to value the person rather than the fat. Consequently, fat talk ("Does this make me look fat?") is not always negative or self-deprecating. It may be a way for people to ask for confirmation *they* have value, whatever their body size.[20] You should give them that validation but avoid equating thinness with beauty and value.
- In some cultural contexts, like Samoa, people have more space to navigate positive as well as negative ideas about their bodies. These spaces of ambivalence are culturally important. We can all help by recognizing and amplifying the positive aspects of being large-bodied (or even, simply, not-thin).
- In some cultural contexts, as in Paraguay and Samoa, it's more acceptable to tease someone about fat, whereas among white people in the United States, there is considerably less face-to-face teasing. Silence in this case does not mean more inclusivity – quite

the opposite. Be aware that context and culture matter, that your social rules do not apply to others, and that stigma can sometimes be more powerful when it is covert.

- In some socioeconomic contexts, like the United States, certain communities feel the effects of obesogenic environments and fat stigma more powerfully than do other communities. Usually, this is because of structural factors. Use an intersectional approach to see how race, ethnicity, and class factors shape who gets sick.
- Be aware that not everyone shares the same understanding of health, illness, and weight. Your understanding may not be the only correct one.

Recommendations for current or future health professionals:

- Don't start clinical encounters with statements like "Let's get the worst part over with," as patients are asked to step on the scales. Patients know and anticipate they are going to be judged biometrically (weight, blood pressure, etc.). Consider not talking about weight, or even weighing the patient, but instead talking about other metrics like blood pressure; think about what kind of interaction you can have that will help the patient's blood pressure be at its most relaxed and thus normal levels. Talk about the weather or season, two topics that most people can discuss with ease (although in agricultural communities this may cause anxiety, so consider the particular norms of the place).
- Remember that the scientific evidence about weight increasingly links environment with weight, making individuals not fully in control of their size. There are a variety of co-occurring conditions that might be more treatable in ways that could have a higher impact on health. For example, treating depression as it relates to diabetes or trauma might be more helpful to your patient. Don't start with weight in your treatment plan.
- Lack of weight loss doesn't mean patients are non-compliant or lazy. Recognize that weight loss might be a priority for people, and people might be emotionally distressed about their weight, but they are balancing multiple other worries and concerns in the everyday contexts of their lives. Ask people about their daily lives. Patients understand that the contexts of their everyday lives often

make it nearly impossible to lose weight, but they don't articulate this. This is a conversation that probably rarely happens in a clinical encounter but should.

- When confronted with medical ideas that are highly fat-negative, many patients react with distrust and rejection toward their doctors and their advice. Temper your judgment, as this will help you keep the trust of your patients.
- Remember that recommending a "healthy diet" is not a neutral statement. The foods people eat every day are shaped by social and economic constraints as well as cultural notions of what makes a meal complete or good.
- Don't make jokes about a fat, sedated patient. The patient may not hear you but the rest of the clinic staff certainly will and they will remember.
- Don't make jokes to or about your fat patient when the clinic infrastructure (gurneys, chairs, needles) can't accommodate them.
- Advocate that your clinic acquires bigger gurneys and chairs. Your population most likely needs them.
- Don't sidestep the entire issue by handing your patient a weight-loss pamphlet at the end of the clinic visit after saying nothing about their weight during the clinic encounter.
- Don't assume your patient is Overweight or Obese; our "eye-ball" assessments are often wrong and shaped by our racial, ethnic, gender, and class-based lens.
- Share these strategies with co-workers and other clinical health professionals.

Recommendations for policy-makers and intervention scientists:

- Large-scale efforts to mobilize public support for efforts to increase exercise and improve eating through individual actions are almost universally doomed to failure. Many of these efforts lead to felt stigma and negative self-sentiments. The data do not support these interventions – they are based on cultural beliefs.
- Helping people learn to identify and move blame into structural challenges should identify more effective points of local intervention. School curricula such as health classes seem a great place to begin. The key here is that all interventions really need to be

locally discussed and defined and they need to focus on structural changes that make sense in people's lives.

- Weight is tied to concerns around social prestige and notions of blame. Subsequently, interventions that focus on weight might be complicating and worsening to health in general and weight management specifically. Avoiding discussions of weight and focusing on health remains the most likely productive strategy as a starting point.
- Gendered patterns of risk of Obesity, in particular, reflect complex but predictable clues about how cultural practices matter for weight risk. For example, in Japan, men are at risk because of the very specific cultural prescriptions around (company) men's work, but women are also affected because they accrue blame for failing to counter it. Make policy that takes gendered risks into account.
- Explicit policies around weight, like the annual metabolic syndrome health examination in Japan, have not proven to be successful (in Japan or elsewhere). They may lead to feelings of shame and drastic disordered eating and behaviors in the few weeks leading up to the health exam. Support those policies that address structural causes of Obesity.
- Implicit policies around weight, like the extra tax placed on sweetened carbonated beverages found in the United States, have not been successful. They appear to result in people feeling shame for their size or their consumption habits. In the case of the sugar tax (in the United States), it tends to hurt those people who lack adequate access to other affordable options. Support those policies that address social disadvantages, rather than policies that are "regressive" or amplify people's disadvantages.

Notes

Foreword

1 Nichter, 2000, p. 37.
2 Nichter, 2000, p. 134.
3 Mendenhall, 2019.
4 Hirsch et al., 2009.
5 Jordan, 1993.
6 Jordan, 1993, p. 4.

1 Introduction

1 Bell, 2016; Crawford, 1980.
2 Bordo, 1993; Greenhalgh, 2016; see also Lester, 2019.
3 Moran-Thomas, 2019, p. 137.
4 Bowen, Brenton, & Elliott, 2019; Langwick, 2018; Roberts, 2017; Yates-Doerr 2015.
5 Gálvez, 2018; Gálvez, Careny, & Yates-Doerr, 2020; Manderson, 2016; Omran, 1971; Popkin, Adair, & Ng, 2012; Popkin & Gordon-Larsen, 2004.
6 Berlant, 2007; Trnka & Trundle, 2017; Rose, 2006.
7 Edmonds, 2010; Gerber, 2012; Griffith, 2004; Garth & Hardin, 2019.
8 Puhl & Brownell, 2006.
9 Brewis, 2014.
10 Karnehed, Rasmussen, Hemmingsson, & Tynelius, 2012; Monteiro, Moura, Conde, & Popkin, 2004; Puhl & Brownell, 2001; Puhl & Heuer, 2010.
11 Puhl & Brownell, 2001.
12 Lee & Pausé, 2016.
13 Greenhalgh & Carney, 2014; Saldaña & Wade, 2018.

14 Brewis & Wutich, 2012.
15 Garth & Hardin, 2019; Yates-Doerr, 2012.
16 Warin & Zivkovic, 2019, p. 162; see also Berlant, 2007.
17 Valdez, 2018.
18 Landecker, 2011; Saldaña-Tejeda, 2017; Saldaña-Tejeda & Wade, 2019; Valdez, 2018; Warin, Moore, Davies, & Ulijaszek, 2016.
19 Valdez, 2018.
20 Sanabria, 2016, p. 135.
21 Brewis, 1996; Brewis & Gartin, 2006; Brewis & McGarvey, 2000; Brewis, McGarvey, Jones, & Swinburn, 1998.
22 Hardin, 2014.
23 Brewis, 2011; Hardin, 2015a, 2015b.
24 L. Miller, 2006.
25 Gartin, 2012.
26 Brewis & Gartin, 2006; see also Baskin, Ard, Franklin, & Allison, 2005; Flegal, Carroll, Kit, & Ogden, 2012; Flegal, Carroll, Kuczmarski, & Johnson, 1998.
27 Brewis, 2003.
28 Trainer, 2017.
29 Trainer, Brewis, & Wutich, 2020; SturtzSreetharan, Trainer, Wutich, & Brewis, 2018; Trainer, Wutich, & Brewis, 2017; Trainer, Brewis, & Wutich, 2017.
30 Agostini, SturtzSreetharan, Wutich, Williams, & Brewis, 2019; SturtzSreetharan, Agostini, Brewis, & Wutich, 2019.
31 Powdermaker, 1960.
32 Becker, 1995; Popenoe, 2004; Sobo, 1994.
33 Carney, 2015; Garth, 2009, 2013, 2020; Hardon & Smith-Morris, 2019; Ikari, 2018; Mendenhall, 2019; Solomon, 2016; Unnithan-Kumar & Tremayne, 2011; Warin & Zivkovic, 2019; Weaver, 2018; Yates-Doerr, 2015.
34 Carney, 2015; Carruth & Mendenhall, 2019.
35 Gálvez, 2018.
36 Mendenhall, 2019.
37 Reese, 2019; Garth & Reese, 2020.
38 Carney, 2015; Garth, 2009, 2013; Hardin, 2015b; Mendenhall, 2016; Mendenhall, Kohrt, Norris, Ndetei, & Prabhakaran, 2017; Solomon, 2016; Trainer, Brewis, Hruschka, & Williams, 2015; Unnithan-Kumar & Tremayne, 2011; Warin & Zivkovic, 2019; Yates-Doerr, 2015.
39 Sanabria, 2016; Sanabria & Yates-Doerr, 2015; Valdez, 2018.
40 Austin, 1999; Gerber, 2012; Hardin, McLennan, & Brewis, 2018; LeBesco, 2011; Lupton, 1993, 2012, 2013; Monaghan, Colls, & Evans, 2013; Puhl, Peterson, & Luedicke, 2013; Sanabria & Yates-Doerr, 2015; Yates-Doerr, 2012.
41 Finucane et al., 2011; Moffat, 2010.
42 Boero, 2013; LeBesco, 2011; Puhl, Peterson, & Luedicke, 2013; Saguy & Almeling, 2008; Saguy & Riley, 2005.

43 Berlant, 2007; Dickinson, 2019; Gálvez, 2018; Gálvez, Carney, & Yates-Doerr, 2020; Kwan, 2009; McNaughton, 2010; Trainer et al., 2017.

44 Brewis & Wutich, 2012; Brewis, Wutich, Falletta-Cowden, & Rodriguez-Soto, 2011; McCullough, 2013; Puhl & Brownell, 2001, 2006; Puhl & Heuer, 2009, 2010.

45 McCullough & Hardin, 2013.

46 Greenhalgh, 2015; Taylor, 2015.

47 Solomon, 2015.

48 Trainer, Brewis, Williams, & Chavez, 2015; Watkins, 2015; Watkins, Farrell, & Hugmeyer, 2012.

49 Alim & Smitherman, 2012.

50 Conrad, 1992, 2005; Salant & Santry, 2006; Stearns, 2002; Wray & Deery, 2008.

51 Rothblum & Solovay, 2009; Saguy & Ward, 2011; Ikari, 2018.

52 Jutel, 2006; Yates-Doerr, 2014.

53 Adams, 2016; Trainer et al., 2015; Yates-Doerr, 2015.

54 Clarke & Haraway, 2018.

55 Brewis, 2014; Brewis, Hruschka, & Wutich, 2011; Edmonds, 2010; Greenhalgh, 2012, 2015, 2016.

56 Anderson-Fye & Brewis, 2017.

57 Forhan & Salas, 2013; Gálvez, 2018; Phelan et al., 2015; Reese, 2018; Schwartz, Chambliss, Brownell, Blair, & Billington, 2003; Taylor, 2011.

58 Trainer et al., 2015.

59 Manderson, 2016; Omran, 1971; Popkin, 1994; Popkin, Adair, & Ng, 2012; Popkin & Gordon-Larsen, 2004.

60 Klingle, 2015; Yates-Doerr, 2015.

61 Moran-Thomas, 2016, 2019.

62 For example, Luke & Cooper, 2013. There is ongoing debate on this point, but the conventional emerging wisdom is that dietary changes are far more influential for weight changes.

63 Sobo, 1994.

64 Roberts, 2015.

65 Solomon, 2016.

66 Trainer, Hardin, SturtzSreetharan, & Brewis, 2020.

67 Burnett, 2018; Ferreira & Lang, 2006; Hoover, 2017; Howard, 2013; Marshall, 2012; McLennan & Ulijaszek, 2015; Mihesuah & Hoover, 2019; Wiedman, 2012.

68 Bell, McNaughton, & Salmon, 2011; Boero, 2012; Counihan & Van Esterik, 2012; Farrell, 2011; Featherstone, 1982; Gimlin, 2002; Greenhalgh, 2016.

69 Bordo, 1993, 2012; Brewis & Wutich, 2019; Groven, 2014; Lester, 2019; Lupton, 2012, 2013; Ogden, Clementi, & Aylwin, 2006; Rubin, Fitts, & Becker, 2003; SturtzSreetharan et al., 2018; Trainer et al., 2017; Warin, 2009.

70 Becker, 2004.

71 Brewis, McGarvey, & Tu`u`au-Potoi, 1998; Brewis, Hruschka, & Wutich, 2011; Brewis & McGarvey, 2000.

72 Miller, 2006.
73 Anderson-Fye & Brewis, 2017.
74 Edmonds, 2010.
75 Popenoe, 2004.
76 Gerber, 2012; Gunson, Warin, & Moore, 2017; Monaghan, 2005; Warin, Turner, Moore, & Davies, 2008; Warin, Zivkovic, Moore, & Davies, 2012.
77 Bourdieu, 1984; Csordas, 1990; Krieger, 2005, 2016; Mauss, 1973.
78 Bordo, 1993; Vogel & Mol, 2014.
79 Rothblum & Solovay, 2009.
80 Boero, 2013; Saguy, 2013.
81 Moffat, 2010, p. 2.
82 Moffat, 2010, p. 2.
83 Greenhalgh & Carney, 2014; Rose & Novas, 2007.
84 Biehl & Petryna, 2013.
85 Brewis, Hruschka, & Wutich, 2011.
86 Bernard, Killworth, Kronenfeld, & Sailer, 1984.

2 How and Where We Did the Study

1   Certainly, this has not always been the case. Anthropology, like most other disciplines, has a long and sordid history. However, more than forty years' worth of debates around decolonizing anthropology and its central practices have produced important self-reflection, critique, and change. See Harrison, 1991; Smith, 2012.
2   Jordan, 1978.
3   Whiting, 1963.
4   Luhrman, Padmavati, Tharoor, & Osei, 2015.
5   Hirsch, Wardlow, & Smith, 2009.
6   Closser et al., 2016.
7   Mendenhall, 2019.
8   Schnegg & Lowe, 2020.
9   Wutich & Brewis, 2019.
10 Hardin, 2015a.
11 We follow anthropologists such as Leith Mullings, Dána-Ain Davis, and Christa Craven and capitalize terms that represent historically marginalized groups, such as Indigenous, Black, Latinx while using lowercase for the term "white" "to decenter whiteness, the racialized identifier that has long served as the norm in disciplines that employ ethnography (Davis & Craven, 2016, p. 4).
12 Brewis, Wutich, Falletta-Cowden, & Rodriguez-Soto, 2011.
13 Brewis & Wutich, 2012.
14 Lunde, 2018.
15 Alvarenga, 2013.
16 Finucane et al., 2011.

17 Finucane et al., 2011; Hodge et al., 1994.
18 Anderson, 2013.
19 Baker, Hanna, & Baker, 1986; Bindon, Crews, & Dressler, 1991; Brewis & McGarvey, 2000; McGarvey, 1992; McGarvey & Baker, 1979.
20 Anae, 2002; Gershon, 2012; Lilomaiava-Doktor, 2009.
21 Hawley et al., 2014; Jaacks et al., 2019.
22 Pollock, 1992.
23 Hodge et al., 1994.
24 Davis & Craven, 2016, p. 9.
25 Gálvez, 2019; Saldaña-Tejeda, 2017; Warin et al., 2008, 2011, 2012; Zivkovic, Warin, Davies, & Moore, 2010.
26 Puhl & Brownell, 2001.
27 Himmelstein, Puhl, & Quinn, 2018, 2019.
28 Berry, Argüelles, Cordis, Ihmoud, & Estrada, 2017.
29 Bejarano, López Juárez, Mijangos García, & Goldstein, 2019; Harrison, 1997; Fabian, 1983; Smith, 1999.
30 Gottlieb, 1995; Yates-Doerr, in press.
31 Behar & Gordon, 1995; Finlay & Gough, 2003; Kondo, 1990; Narayan, 1993; Navarro, Williams, & Ahmad, 2013; Wolf, 1996.
32 Reiter & Rapp, 1975; Rosaldo & Lamphere, 1974; Weiner, 1976.
33 Reiter & Rapp, 1975; Rosaldo & Lamphere, 1974; Weiner, 1976.
34 Wolf, 1996.
35 Geertz, 1988.
36 Craven & Davis, 2013; Davis & Craven, 2016; El Kotni, Dixon, & Miranda, 2020; Lutz, 1990.
37 Warin & Gunson, 2013.
38 See Hardin, 2019, for a discussion of "radical listening."

3 *Futotteru* (Fat) in Osaka, Japan

1 *Jisho, Japanese-English Dictionary*, s.v. "kuidaore," https://jisho.org/search/kuidaore.
2 Wakita, 1999.
3 Inoue, Takamiya, Yoshiike, & Shimomitsu, 2006.
4 In the United States, the average is 5,117 steps a day; in Australia, 9,695 steps; in Switzerland, 9,650 steps; and in Japan, 7,168 steps. See Bassett et al., 2010.
5 Brewis, Trainer, Han, & Wutich, 2017; Colls & Evans, 2014; Garland, 2011; Livingston, 2000.
6 Umeda Station, located in Osaka and conjoined with Osaka Station, is the fourth busiest in the world as measured by number of travelers who use the station on a daily basis. See Blaster, 2013.
7 Traphagan and Brown argue that eating out at fast food establishments is not only about convenience and harried urban lives. They suggest that

"fast food-establishments in Japan express, facilitate, and strengthen traditional patterns of intergenerational commensality." See Traphagan & Brown, 2002, p. 120.

8 Yoshinoya is one of the oldest fast food restaurants in Japan, operating since 1899. It has restaurants in Japan and in the United States (https://www.yoshinoya.com/en/).

9 This is the only section of the text where we use the terms "obesity" and "overweight" rather than the term "fat." As we point out in the introduction, fat tends to be the preferred term among many critical scholars writing today, and obesity and overweight tend to be viewed as problematic by many social scientists. However, Obesity and over-weight are still the common rubric used by most public health entities, as are BMI measurements. The recent public health measures undertaken by the Japanese government are all couched in this terminology and, thus, to discuss the measures, we necessarily need to reference the terms.

10 As an example, see Miller, 2016. See also a report issued by WHO, 2004.

11 Hruschka and Hadley discuss the problems with using BMI (which is based on weight and height) as a means of measuring and comparing body fat across populations. See Hruschka & Hadley, 2016.

12 Government of Japan, Ministry of Health, Labor and Welfare, 2020.

13 Tanaka & Kinoshita, 2009, p. 6.

14 Manzenreiter, 2012, p. 69.

15 Mah, 2010, p. 393; Takeda & Melby, 2017; Takeda, Melby, & Ishikawa, 2017.

16 Borovoy, 2017.

17 Borovoy, 2017.

18 Allison, 2003.

19 For a similar discussion around men's alcohol addiction in Japan, see Borovoy, 2005.

20 Castro-Vázquez, 2020.

21 Alexy, 2007; Borovoy, 2005, 2017; Pike & Borovoy, 2004.

22 Tanaka, Itō, & Hattori, 2002.

23 See Miller, 2006.

24 This imprecision was noted by Mimi Nichter in the US context twenty years ago. See Nichter, 2000.

25 Cwiertka, 2006; Takeda, 2008.

26 See Ohnuki-Tierny, 1993.

27 Takeda et al., 2018.

28 A commonly observed phenomenon is that the fat body becomes open to public commentary.

29 Dasgupta, 2003; North, 2009.

30 Farrell, 2011; Gard & Wright, 2005; Lee & Pausé, 2016; Namate, Saito, & Sawamiya, 2016.

31 In an exercise investigating impressions of personality traits with body shape, very thin Japanese female figures were the least likely to be rated favorably. See Namate et al., 2016.
32 Katare & Beatty, 2018.

4 Fat in Peri-rural Georgia, USA

1 Buer, Leukefeld, & Havens, 2016; Raskin, 2015, 2017; Welch, 2014.
2 Community Farm Alliance, n.d.; Center of Appalachian Studies & Services, n.d.; Curtis, 2017; Humiston, 2015; Jaschik, 2014; Raskin, 2015, 2017.
3 Cottom, 2019; Gay, 2017; Laymon, 2018; McClure, 2013; Patterson-Faye, 2016; Strings, 2019.
4 Ogden, Carroll, Fryar, & Flegal, 2015; Ogden, Lamb, Carroll, & Flegal, 2010; Ogden, Carroll, Brian, & Flegal, 2014; State of Childhood Obesity, n.d.; Wolfe, 2017a, 2017b.
5 SturtzSreetharan, Trainer, Wutich, & Brewis, 2018; Trainer et al., 2017; Trainer et al., 2017; Trainer, Brewis, Hruschka et al., 2015; Trainer, Brewis, Wutich, Kurtz, & Niesluchowski, 2016.
6 Becker, 1995; Boero, 2010, 2012; Bordo, 1993, 2012; Braziel & Lebesco, 2001; Brewis, 2014; Farrell, 2011; McCullough & Hardin, 2013; Puhl & Heuer, 2009, 2010; Rogge, 2004; Rothblum & Solovay, 2009; Scheper-Hughes & Lock, 1987; Shafer, 1991; Turner, 1982, 1984; Weber, 2002; Zigon, 2008.
7 Calogero, Tylka, & Mensinger, 2016; Chrisler, 2012; Fikkan & Rothblum, 2012; Saguy, 2012.
8 Becker, 1995; Boero, 2010, 2012; Bordo, 1993, 2012; Braziel & Lebesco, 2001; Brewis, 2014; Farrell, 2011; McCullough & Hardin, 2013; Puhl & Heuer, 2009, 2010; Rogge, 2004; Rothblum & Solovay, 2009; Scheper-Hughes & Lock, 1987; Shafer, 1991; Turner, 1982, 1984; Weber, 2002; Zigon, 2008.

5 *Gordura* (Fat) in Encarnación, Paraguay

1 Oldani & Baigún, 2002.
2 IPS Correspondents, 2008.
3 Coen, Ross, & Turner, 2008.
4 Catholic News Agency, 2015, para. 24.
5 Romero, 2012.
6 Lambert & Nickson, 2013.
7 Folch, 2012.
8 Knoema, 2016.
9 World Health Organization, 2016.
10 Ultima Hora, 2011.
11 Geggel, 2017.

12 *Piropos* can also be simple whistles or catcalls – sometimes offensive, disgusting, or frightening. For this reason, one woman told Amber, there have been efforts to outlaw *piropos* in Encarnación, and one hears them less often on the street these days.

6 *Lapoʻa* (Large) in Apia, Samoa

1 Samoan Bureau of Statistics, 2011.
2 Macpherson & Macpherson, 2010.
3 Gershon, 2000.
4 Kahn, 1986; Malinowski, 1925; Young, 1972.
5 Keighley et al., 2007; Singer, 2014; Snowdon & Thow, 2013.
6 Choy et al., 2017.
7 Anderson, 2013; Hawley & McGarvey, 2015.
8 Finucane et al., 2011.
9 Hawley et al., 2014.
10 Hardin & Kwauk, 2019.
11 Hardin & Kwauk, 2019, p. 382.
12 Field, 2012, paras. 6, 7.
13 Gewertz & Errington, 2010.
14 Farmer, 2003.

7 The Bigger Picture: Shared Beliefs about Fat

1 Chalkin, 2016; Hole, 2003; Nichols, Lewis, & Shreves, 2015.
2 Brewis & Gartin, 2006; Mendenhall, 2019.
3 Castro-Vázquez (2020) talks about this as the "ethnicized veiwpoint of corpulence" that is common in Japan, especially visible in Japan's metabolic health policies.

8 Conclusions: A Global Perspective on Weight

1 Brewis, 2011; McCullough & Hardin, 2013.
2 Nestle, 2007.
3 Brewis, 2014; Tomiyama et al., 2018.
4 McCullough & Hardin, 2013.
5 Dionne, 2019; "Fat activism," n.d.; Seversen, 2019; Thompson, 2017; Tovar, 2019; Trainer, Brewis, Williams et al., 2015.

Appendices

1 SturtzSreetharan, 2004, 2006, 2009, 2017.
2 Brewis, SturtzSreetharan, & Wutich, 2018; SturtzSreetharan & Brewis, 2019; SturtzSreetharan, Trainer, Wutich, & Brewis, 2018.

3 Brewis, 2011; Brewis & Wutich, 2015; Brewis & Wutich, 2019; Brewis, Wutich, Falletta-Cowden, & Rodriguez-Soto, 2011.

4 Brewis, 1996, 2003; Brewis & Gartin, 2006; Brewis, McGarvey, Jones, & Swinburn, 1998.

5 Brewis, 2011.

6 Hardin, 2019.

7 Hardin, 2013, 2016, 2018.

8 Hardin & Kwauk, 2015, 2019.

9 Trainer, 2013, 2017.

10 Trainer, Brewis, Williams et al., 2015.

11 Trainer et al., 2017

12 Trainer et al., 2016.

13 Wutich, Roberts, White, Larson, & Brewis, 2014.

14 Brewis et al., 2018.

15 Heaton, 2004.

16 Tracy, 2010.

17 Guest, Bunce, & Johnson, 2006; Hagaman & Wutich, 2017.

18 Bernard, Wutich, & Ryan, 2016.

19 Bernard et al., 2016; MacQueen, McLellan, Kelly, & Milstein, 1998.

20 Agostini et al., 2019; SturtzSreetharan et al., 2019.

References

Adams, V. (2016). *Metrics: What counts in global health*. Durham, NC: Duke University Press.

Agostini, G., SturtzSreetharan, C., Wutich, A., Williams, D., & Brewis, A. (2019). Citizen sociolinguistics: A new method for understanding fat talk and other sociolinguistic phenomena. *PLOS One, 14*(5), e0217618.

Alexy, A. (2007). Deferred benefits, romance, and the specter of later-life divorce. *Contemporary Japan, 19*(1), 169–88.

Alim, S., & Smitherman, G. (2012). *Articulate while Black: Barack Obama, language, and race in the US*. New York, NY: Oxford University Press.

Allison, A. (2013). Japanese mothers and obentōs: The lunch-box as ideological state apparatus. In C. Counihan & P. Van Esterik (Eds.), *Food and culture: A reader* (pp. 154–72). New York, NY: Taylor and Francis.

Alvarenga, D.B. (2013). *Terere* as a social bond. In P. Lambert & A. Nickson (Eds.), *The Paraguay reader: History, culture, politics* (pp. 426–32). Durham, NC: Duke University Press.

Anae, M. (2002). Papalagi redefined: Towards a NZ-born Samoan identity. In P. Spickard (Ed.), *Pacific diaspora: Island peoples in the United States and across the Pacific* (pp. 150–69). Honolulu, HI: University of Hawai'i Press.

Anderson, I. (2013). The economic costs of non-communicable diseases in the Pacific Islands: A rapid stock take of the situation in Samoa, Tonga, and Vanuatu. The World Bank. Discussion paper 86522. http://documents.worldbank.org/curated/en/291471468063255184/The-economic-costs-of-non-communicable-diseases-in-the-Pacific-Islands-a-rapid-stock-take-of-the-situation-in-Samoa-Tonga-and-Vanuatu

Anderson-Fye, E.P., & Brewis, A. (Eds.). (2017). *Fat planet: Obesity, culture, and symbolic body capital*. Santa Fe, NM: School of American Research Press.

Austin, S.B. (1999). Fat, loathing and public health: The complicity of science in a culture of disordered eating. *Culture, Medicine and Psychiatry, 23*(2), 245–68.

Baker, P.T., Hanna, J.M., & Baker, T.S. (1986). *The changing Samoans: Behavior and health in transition.* New York, NY: Oxford University Press.

Baskin, M.L., Ard, J., Franklin, F., & Allison, D.B. (2005). Prevalence of obesity in the United States. *Obesity Reviews, 6*(1), 5–7.

Bassett, D.R. Jr., Wyatt, H., Thompson, H., Peters, J., & Hill, J. (2010). Pedometer-measured physical activity and health behaviors in U.S. adults. *Medicine & Science in Sports & Exercise, 42*(10), 1819–25. doi: 10.1249 /MSS.0b013e3181dc2e54.

Becker, A.E. (1995). *Body, self and society: The view from Fiji.* Philadelphia, PA: University of Pennsylvania Press.

Becker, A.E. (2004). Television, disordered eating, and young women in Fiji: Negotiating body image and identity during rapid social change. *Culture Medicine & Psychiatry, 28*(4), 533–59.

Behar, R., & Gordon, D. (1995). *Women writing culture.* Berkeley, CA: University of California Press.

Bejarano, C.A., López Juárez, L., Mijangos García, M., & Goldstein, D. (2019). *Decolonizing ethnography: Undocumented immigrants and new directions in social science.* Durham, NC: Duke University Press.

Bell, K. (2016). *Health and other unassailable values: Reconfigurations of health, evidence and ethics.* New York, NY: Taylor & Francis.

Bell, K., McNaughton, D., & Salmon, A. (Eds.). (2011). *Alcohol, tobacco, and obesity: Morality, mortality, and the new public health.* London, UK: Routledge.

Berlant, L. (2007). Slow death (sovereignty, obesity, lateral agency). *Critical Inquiry, 33*(4), 754–80.

Bernard, H.R., Killworth, P.D., Kronenfeld, D., & Sailer, L. (1984). The problem of informant accuracy: The validity of retrospective data. *Annual Review of Anthropology, 13*, 495–517.

Bernard, H.R., Wutich, A., & Ryan, G. (2016). *Analyzing qualitative data: Systematic approaches.* Thousand Oaks, CA: Sage.

Berry, M.J., Argüelles, C.C., Cordis, S., Ihmoud, S., & Estrada, E.V. (2017). Toward a fugitive anthropology: Gender, race, and violence in the field. *Cultural Anthropology, 32*(4), 537–65.

Biehl, J., & Petryna, A. (2013). *When people come first: Critical studies in global health.* Princeton, NJ: Princeton University Press.

Bindon, J., Crews, D.E., & Dressler, W.W. (1991). Life style, modernization and adaptation among Samoans. *Collegium Antropolgicum, 15*(1), 101–10.

Blaster, M. (2013). The 51 busiest train stations in the world – All but 6 located in Japan. *Japan Today,* 6 February. https://japantoday.com/category /features/travel/the-51-busiest-train-stations-in-the-world-all-but-6 -located-in-japan

Boero, N. (2010). Bypassing blame: Bariatric surgery and the case of biomedical failure. In L. Mamo, A.E. Clarke, J.R. Fosket, J.R. Fishman, & J.K. Shim (Eds.), *Biomedicalization: Technoscience, health and illness in the U.S.* (pp. 307–30). Durham, NC: Duke University Press.

Boero, N. (2012). *Killer fat: Media, medicine, and morals in the American "obesity epidemic."* New Brunswick, NJ: Rutgers University Press.

Boero, N. (2013). Obesity in the media: Social science weighs in. *Critical Public Health, 23*(3), 371–80.

Bordo, S. (1993). *Unbearable weight: Feminism, Western culture, and the body.* Berkeley, CA: University of California Press.

Bordo, S. (2012). Not just "a White girl's thing": The changing face of food and body image problems. In C. Counihan & P. Van Esterik (Eds.), *Food and culture: A reader* (3rd ed.) (pp. 265–75). New York, NY: Routledge.

Borovoy, A. (2005). *The too-good wife: Alcohol, codependence, and the politics of nurturance in postwar Japan.* Berkeley, CA: University of California Press.

Borovoy, A. (2017). Japan's public health paradigm: Governmentality and the containment of harmful behavior. *Medical Anthropology, 36*(1), 32–46.

Bourdieu, P. (1984). *Distinction: A social critique of the judgement of taste.* Cambridge, MA: Harvard University Press.

Bowen, S., Brenton, J., & Elliott, S. (2019). *Pressure cooker: Why home cooking won't solve our problems and what we can do about it.* New York, NY: Oxford University Press.

Braziel, J.E., & Lebesco, K. (Eds.). (2001). *Bodies out of bounds.* Berkeley, CA: University of California Press.

Brewis, A. (1996). *Lives on the line: Women and ecology on a Pacific atoll.* Fort Worth, TX: Harcourt Brace College Publishers.

Brewis, A. (2003). Biocultural aspects of obesity in young Mexican schoolchildren. *American Journal of Human Biology, 15*(3), 446–60.

Brewis, A. (2011). *Obesity: Cultural and biocultural perspectives.* New Brunswick, NJ: Rutgers University Press.

Brewis, A. (2014). Stigma and the perpetuation of obesity. *Social Science & Medicine, 118*, 152–8.

Brewis, A., & Gartin, M. (2006). Biocultural constructions of obesogenic ecologies of childhood: Parental feeding versus young child eating strategies. *American Journal of Human Biology, 18*, 203–13.

Brewis, A., Hruschka, D., & Wutich, A. (2011). Vulnerability to fat-stigma in women's everyday relationships. *Social Science & Medicine, 73*(4), 491–7.

Brewis, A., & McGarvey, S. (2000). Body image, body size and Samoan ecological and individual modernization. *Ecology of Food and Nutrition, 39*(2), 105–20.

Brewis, A., McGarvey, S., Jones, J., & Swinburn, B. (1998). Perceptions of body size in Pacific Islanders. *International Journal of Obesity, 22*(2), 185–9.

Brewis, A., McGarvey, S., & Tu'u'au-Potoi, N. (1998). Structure of family planning in Samoa. *Australian Journal of Public Health, 22*(4), 424–7. https://doi.org/10.1111/j.1467-842X.1998.tb01407.x

Brewis, A., SturtzSreetharan, C., & Wutich, A. (2018). Obesity stigma as a global health challenge. *Globalization and Health, 14*, 20.

Brewis, A., Trainer, S., Han, S.Y., & Wutich, A. (2017). Publicly misfitting: Extreme weight and the everyday production and reinforcement of felt stigma. *Medical Anthropology Quarterly, 31*(2), 257–76.

Brewis, A., & Wutich, A. (2012). Explicit versus implicit fat-stigma. *American Journal of Human Biology: The Official Journal of the Human Biology Council, 24*(3), 332–8. https://doi.org/10.1002/ajhb.22233

Brewis, A., & Wutich, A. (2015). A world of suffering? Fat stigma in the global contexts of the obesity epidemic. In T. Leatherman (Ed.), Critical biocultural approaches to health disparities. Special issue of *Annals of Anthropological Practice, 38*, 271–85.

Brewis, A., & Wutich, A. (2019). *Lazy, crazy, and disgusting: Stigma and the undoing of public health.* Baltimore, MD: Johns Hopkins University Press.

Brewis, A., Wutich, A., Falletta-Cowden, A., & Rodriguez-Soto, I. (2011). Body norms and fat stigma in global perspective. *Current Anthropology, 52*(2), 269–76.

Buer, L.M., Leukefeld, C.G., & Havens, J.R. (2016). "I'm stuck": Women's navigations of social networks and prescription drug misuse in central Appalachia. *North American Dialogue, 19*(2), 70–84.

Burnett, D. (2018). *Migrant indigeneity: Transnational health policy implementation structuring the body, identity, & belief* [Unpublished doctoral dissertation]. University of Pennsylvania.

Calogero, R.M., Tylka, T.L., & Mensinger, J.L. (2016). Scientific weightism: A view of mainstream weight stigma research through a feminist lens. In T.A. Roberts, N. Curtin, L.E. Duncan, & L.M. Cortina (Eds.), *Feminist perspectives on building a better psychological science of gender* (pp. 9–28). Zurich, Switzerland: Springer International Publishing.

Carney, M. (2015). *The unending hunger: Tracing women and food insecurity across borders.* Berkeley, CA: University of California Press.

Carruth, L., & Mendenhall, E. (2019). "Wasting away": Diabetes, food insecurity, and medical insecurity in the Somali region of Ethiopia. *Social Science & Medicine, 228*, 155–63.

Castro-Vázquez, G. (2020). *Masculinity and body weight in Japan: Grappling with metabolic syndrome.* New York, NY: Routledge.

Catholic News Agency. (2015). *Happiness and pleasure are not synonyms, Pope Francis reminds Paraguay's youth.* CNA, 11 July. https://www.catholicnewsagency.com/news/happiness-and-pleasure-are-not-synonyms-pope-francis-reminds-paraguays-youth-70975

Center of Appalachian Studies & Services. (n.d.). *Appalachian teaching project.* CASS. Accessed 9 December 2020. http://www.etsu.edu/cas/cass/projects/

Chalkin, V. (2016). Obstinate fatties: Fat activism, queer negativity, and the celebration of "obesity." *Subjectivity, 9*, 107–25.

Choy, C.C., Desai, M.M., Park, J.J., Frame, E.A., Thompson, A.A., Naseri, T., ... & Hawley, N.L. (2017). Child, maternal and household-level correlates of nutritional status: A cross-sectional study among young Samoan children. *Public Health Nutrition, 20*(7), 1235–47.

Chrisler, J.C. (2012). "Why can't you control yourself?" Fat should be a feminist issue. *Sex Roles, 66*, 608–16.

Clarke, A., & Haraway, D. (2018). *Making kin not population.* Chicago, IL: Prickly Paradigm Press.

Closser, S., Rosenthal, A., Maes, K., Justice, J., Cox, K., Omidian, P., Mohammed, I.Z., Dukku, A.M., Koon, A.D., & Nyirazinyoye, L. (2016). The global context of vaccine refusal: Insights from a systematic comparative ethnography of the global polio eradication initiative. *Medical Anthropology Quarterly, 30*(3), 321–41.

Coen, S.E., Ross, N.A., & Turner, S. (2008). "Without tiendas it's a dead neighbourhood": The socio-economic importance of small trade stores in Cochabamba, Bolivia. *Cities, 25*(6), 327–39.

Colls, R., & Evans, B. (2014). Making space for fat bodies? A critical account of "the obesogenic environment." *Progress in Human Geography, 38*(6), 733–53.

Community Farm Alliance (CFA). (n.d.). *Breaking beans: The Appalachian food story project.* CFA. Accessed 9 December 2020. https://cfaky.org/programs/breaking-beans-the-appalachian-food-story-project/

Conrad, P. (1992). Medicalization and social control. *Annual Review of Sociology, 18*, 209–32.

Conrad, P. (2005). The shifting engines of medicalization. *Journal of Health and Social Behavior, 46*(1), 3–14.

Cottom, T.M. (2019). *Thick and other essays.* New York, NY: The New Press.

Counihan, C., & Van Esterik, P. (Eds.). (2012). *Food and culture: A reader* (3rd ed.). New York, NY: Routledge.

Craven, C., & Davis, D. (2013). *Feminist activist ethnography: Counterpoints to new liberalism in North America.* New York, NY: Rowman & Littlefield.

Crawford, R. (1980). Healthism and the medicalization of everyday life. *International Journal of Health Services, 10*, 365–88.

Csordas, T.J. (1990). Embodiment as a paradigm for anthropology. *Ethos, 18*(1), 5–47.

Curtis, K. (2017). *Breaking beans: Food before it was a "system."* Community Farm Alliance. https://cfaky.org/2017/01/18/food-before-it-was-a-system/

Cwiertka, K. (2006). *Modern Japanese cuisine: Food, power, and national identity.* London, UK: Reaktion Books.

Dasgupta, R. (2003). Creating corporate warriors: The "salaryman" and masculinity in Japan. In K. Louie & M. Low (Eds.), *Asian masculinities: The meaning and practice of manhood in China and Japan* (pp. 118–34). London, UK: RoutledgeCurzon.

Davis, D., & Craven, C. (2016). *Feminist ethnography: Thinking through methodologies, challenges and possibilities*. New York, NY: Rowman & Littlefield.

Dickinson, M. (2019). *Feeding the crisis: Care and abandonment in America's food safety net*. Oakland, CA: University of California Press.

Dionne, E. (2019). Here's what fat acceptance is – and isn't. *YES! Magazine*, 24 June. https://www.yesmagazine.org/social-justice/2019/06/24/fat-acceptance-movement/

Edmonds, A. (2010). *Pretty modern: Beauty, sex, and plastic surgery in Brazil*. Durham, NC: Duke University Press.

El Kotni, M., Dixon, L.Z., & Miranda, V. (2020). Co-authorship as feminist writing and practice. *Society for Cultural Anthropology*, 6 February. https://culanth.org/fieldsights/series/co-authorship-as-feminist-writing-and-practice-1

Fabian, J. (1983). *Time and the other: How anthropology makes its object*. New York, NY: Columbia University Press.

Farmer, P. (2003). *Pathologies of power: Health, human rights, and the new war on the poor*. Berkeley, CA: University of California Press.

Farrell, A. (2011). *Fat shame: Stigma and the fat body in American culture*. New York, NY: New York University Press.

Fat Activism. (n.d.). Charlotte talks with Mike Collins. LiveRadio WFAE. Accessed 9 December 2020. https://www.wfae.org/post/fat-activism#stream/0

Featherstone, M. (1982). The body in consumer culture. *Theory, Culture, & Society, 1*(2), 18–33.

Ferreira, M., & Lang, G. (2006). *Indigenous peoples and diabetes: Community empowerment and wellness*. Durham, NC: Carolina Academic Press.

Field, M. (2012). Samoa's poor are "lazy": PM Stuff.co, 24 January. http://www.stuff.co.nz/world/6305942/Samoa-s-poor-are-lazy-PM

Fikkan, J.L., & Rothblum, E.D. (2012). Is fat a feminist issue? Exploring the gendered nature of weight bias. *Sex Roles, 66*, 575–92.

Finlay, L., & Gough, B. (Eds.). (2003). *Reflexivity: A practical guide for researchers*. Oxford, UK: Blackwell Publishing.

Finucane, M.M., Stevens, G.A., Cowan, M.J., Danaei, G., Lin, J.K., Paciorek, C.J., ... & Global Burden of Metabolic Risk Factors of Chronic Diseases Collaborating Group (BMI). (2011). National, regional, and global trends in body-mass index since 1980: Systematic analysis of health examination surveys and epidemiological studies with 960 country-years and 9.1 million participants. *Lancet, 377*(9765), 557–67.

Flegal, K.M., Carroll, M.D., Kit, B.K., & Ogden, C.L. (2012). Prevalence of obesity and trends in the distribution of body mass index among US adults, 1999–2010. *Jama, 307*(5), 491–7.

Flegal, K.M., Carroll, M.D., Kuczmarski, R.J., & Johnson, C.L. (1998). Overweight and obesity in the United States: Prevalence and trends, 1960–1994. *International Journal of Obesity, 22*(1), 39.

Folch, C. (2012). Trouble on the triple frontier. *Foreign Affairs*, 6 September. https://www.foreignaffairs.com/articles/argentina/2012-09-06/trouble -triple-frontier

Forhan, M., & Salas, X.R. (2013). Inequities in health care: A review of bias and discrimination in obesity treatment. *Canadian Journal of Diabetes*, 37(3), 205–9. https://doi.org/10.1016/j.jcjd.2013.03.362

Gálvez, A. (2018). *Eating NAFTA: Trade, food policies, and the destruction of Mexico*. Berkeley, CA: University of California Press.

Gálvez, A. (2019).Transnational mother blame: Protecting and caring in a globalized context. *Medical Anthropology, 38*(7), 574–87.

Gálvez, A., Carney, M., & Yates-Doerr, E. (2020). Chronic disaster: Reimagining noncommunicable chronic disease. *American Anthropologist*, 122(3), 639–40.

Gard, M., & Wright, J. (2005). *The obesity epidemic: Science, morality, and ideology*. New York, NY: Routledge.

Garland, T.R. (2011). Misfits: A feminist materialist disability concept. *Hypatia, 26*(3), 591–609.

Garth, H. (2009). "Things became scarce": Food availability and accessibility in Santiago de Cuba then and now. *NAPA Bulletin, 32*, 178–92.

Garth, H. (2013). Obesity in Cuba: Memories of the special period and approaches to weight loss today. In M. McCullough & J. Hardin (Eds.), *Reconstructing obesity: The measures of meaning, the meaning of measures* (pp. 89–106). New York, NY: Berghahn Books.

Garth, H. (2020). *Food in Cuba: The pursuit of a decent meal*. Stanford, CA: Stanford University Press.

Garth, H., & Hardin, J. (2019). On the limitations of barriers: Social visibility and weight management in Cuba and Samoa. *Social Science & Medicine, 239*, 112501.

Garth, H., & Reese, A.M. (2020). *Black food matters: Racial justice in the wake of food justice*. Minneapolis, MN: University of Minnesota Press.

Gartin, M. (2012). Food deserts and nutritional risk in Paraguay. *American Journal of Human Biology, 24*(3), 296–301.

Gay, R. (2017). *Hunger: A memoir of (my) body*. New York, NY: HarperCollins.

Geertz, C. (1988). *Works and lives: The anthropologist as author*. Stanford, CA: Stanford University Press.

Geggel, L. (2017). This country, once again, is the happiest nation in the world. *Live Science*. https://www.livescience.com/59633-2017-report-on-world -happiness.html

Gerber, L. (2012). *Seeking the straight and narrow: Weight loss and sexual reorientation in evangelical America*. Chicago, IL: University of Chicago Press.

Gershon, I. (2000). How to know when not to know: Strategic ignorance when eliciting for Samoan migrant exchanges. *Social Analysis 44*(2), 84–105.

Gershon, I. (2012). *No family is an island: Cultural expertise among Samoans in diaspora*. Ithaca, NY: Cornell University Press.

Gewertz, D., & Errington, F. (2010). *Cheap meat: Flap food nations in the Pacific Islands*. Berkeley, CA: University of California Press.

Gimlin, D. (2002). *Body work: Beauty and self-image in American culture*. Berkeley, CA: University of California Press.

Gottlieb, A. (1995). Beyond the lonely anthropologist: Collaboration in research and writing. *American Anthropologist, 97*, 21–6.

Government of Japan, Ministry of Health, Labor and Welfare. (2020, January 14). Heisei 30 nen: Kokumin kenkō, eiyō chōsa kekka gaiyōu [Heisei year 30: Summary of national health and nutrition survey]. https://www.mhlw.go.jp/stf/newpage_08789.html

Greenhalgh, S. (2012). Weighty subjects: The biopolitics of the US war on fat. *American Ethnologist, 39*(3), 471–87.

Greenhalgh, S. (2015). *Fat-talk nation: The human costs of America's war on fat*. Ithaca, NY: Cornell University Press.

Greenhalgh, S. (2016). Disordered eating/eating disorder: Hidden perils of the nation's fight against fat. *Medical Anthropology Quarterly, 30*(4), 545–62. https://doi.org/10.1111/maq.12257

Greenhalgh, S., & Carney, M. (2014). Bad biocitizens? Latinos and the US "obesity epidemic." *Human Organization, 73*(3), 267–76.

Griffith, R.M. (2004). *Born again bodies: Flesh and spirit in American Christianity*. Berkeley, CA: University of California Press.

Groven, K. (2014). They think surgery is just a quick fix. *International Journal of Qualitative Studies on Health and Well-Being, 9*. doi: 10.3402/qhw.v9.24378

Guest, G., Bunce, A., & Johnson, L. (2006). How many interviews are enough? An experiment with data saturation & variability. *Field Methods, 18*(1), 59–82.

Gunson, J.S., Warin, M., & Moore, V. (2017). Visceral politics: Obesity and children's embodied experiences of food and hunger. *Critical Public Health, 27*(4), 407–18.

Hagaman, A., & Wutich, A. (2017). How many interviews are enough to identify metathemes in multisited and cross-cultural research? Another perspective on Guest, Bunce, and Johnson's (2006) Landmark Study. *Field Methods, 29*(1), 23–41.

Hardin, J. (2013). Fasting for health, fasting for God: Samoan evangelical Christian responses to obesity and chronic disease. In M. McCullough & J. Hardin (Eds.), *Reconstructing obesity: The measures of meaning, the meaning of measures* (pp. 107–30). New York, NY: Berghahn Books.

Hardin, J. (2014). *Spiritual etiologies: Metabolic disorders, evangelical Christianity, and well-being in Samoa* [Unpublished doctoral dissertation]. Brandeis University.

Hardin, J. (2015a). Christianity, fat talk, and Samoan pastors: Rethinking the fat-positive-fat-stigma framework. *Fat Studies: An Interdisciplinary Journal of Body Weight and Society, 4*(2), 178–96.

Hardin, J. (2015b). Everyday translation: Health practitioners' perspectives on obesity and metabolic disorders in Samoa. *Critical Public Health, 25*(2), 125–38.

Hardin, J. (2016). "Healing is a done deal": Temporality and metabolic healing among evangelical Christians in Samoa. *Medical Anthropology,* *35*(2), 105–18. https://doi.org/10.1080/01459740.2015.1092143

Hardin, J. (2018). Embedded narratives: Metabolic disorders and Pentecostal conversion in Samoa. *Medical Anthropology Quarterly, 32*(1), 22–41.

Hardin, J. (2019). *Faith and the pursuit of health: Cardiometabolic disorders in Samoa.* New Brunswick, NJ: Rutgers University Press.

Hardin, J., & Kwauk, C.T. (2015). Producing markets, producing people: Local food, financial prosperity and health in Samoa. *Food, Culture & Society, 18*(3), 519–39. https://doi.org/10.1080/15528014.2015.1043113

Hardin, J., & Kwauk, C.T. (2019). Elemental eating: Samoan public health and valuation. *The Contemporary Pacific, 3*(2), 381–415. doi: 10.1353/cp.2019.0027

Hardin, J., McLennan, A.K., & Brewis, A. (2018). Body size, body norms and some unintended consequences of obesity intervention in the Pacific Islands. *Annals of Human Biology, 45*(3), 285–94. https://doi.org/10.1080/03014460.2018.1459838

Hardon, A., & Smith-Morris, C. (2019). Reconfiguring metabolism: Critical ethnographies of obesity and diabetes. *Medical Anthropology, 38*(8), 777–80.

Harrison, F. (Ed.). (1991). *Decolonizing anthropology: Moving further toward and anthropology for liberation.* Washington, DC: American Anthropological Association.

Harrison, F. (Ed.). (1997). *Decolonizing anthropology: Moving further toward an anthropology for liberation* (2nd ed.). Arlington, VA: American Anthropological Association.

Hawley, N.L., & McGarvey, S. (2015). Obesity and diabetes in Pacific Islanders: The current burden and the need for urgent action. *Current Diabetes Reports, 15*(5), 1–10.

Hawley, N.L., Minster, R.L., Weeks, D.E., Viali, S., Reupena, M.S., Sun, G., ... & McGarvey, S. (2014). Prevalence of adiposity and associated cardiometabolic risk factors in the Samoan genome-wide association study. *American Journal of Human Biology, 26*(4), 491–501. https://doi.org/10.1002/ajhb.22553

Heaton, J. (2004). *Reworking qualitative data.* Thousand Oaks, CA: Sage.

Himmelstein, M., Puhl, R., & Quinn, D. (2018). Weight stigma in men: What, when, and by whom? *Obesity, 26,* 968–76.

Himmelstein, M., Puhl, R., & Quinn, D. (2019). Overlooked and understudied: Health consequences of weight stigma in men. *Obesity, 27*(10), 1598–605. doi:10.1002/oby.22599

Hirsch, J.S., Wardlow, H., Smith, D.J., Phinney, H., Parikh, S., & Nathanson, C. (2009). *The secret: Love, marriage, and HIV.* Nashville, TN: Vanderbilt University Press.

Hodge, A.M., Dowse, G.K., Toelupe, P., Collins, V.R., Imo, T., & Zimmet, V.R. (1994). Dramatic increase in the prevalence of obesity in Western Samoa over the 13 year period 1978–1991. *International Journal of Obesity, 18,* 419–28.

Hole, A. (2003). Performing identity: Dawn French and the funny fat female body. *Feminist Media Studies, 3*(3), 315–28.

Hoover, E. (2017). *The river is in us: Fighting toxics in a Mohawk community.* Minneapolis, MN: University of Minnesota Press.

Howard, H.A. (2013). Canadian residential schools and urban Indigenous knowledge production about diabetes. *Medical Anthropology, 33*(6), 529–45.

Hruschka, D., & Hadley, C. (2016). How much do universal anthropometric standards bias the global monitoring of obesity and undernutrition? *Obesity Review, 17*(11), 1030–9.

Humiston, M. (Ed.). (2015). *Community Farm Alliance 2014–2015 – Breaking beans: The Appalachian food story project final report.* Community Farm Alliance, Blue Moon Fund, and the Chorus Foundation. https://cfaky.org/wp-content/uploads/2018/01/breaking-beans-report-final-with-stories.pdf

Ikari, Y. (2018). *"Fatto" no minzokushi: Gendai amerika ni okeru himan mondai to sei no tayōsei.* [Ethnogrophy of "fat": Obesity epidemic and diversity in the United States.] Tokyo, Japan: Akashi Shoten.

Inoue, S., Takamiya, T., Yoshiike, N., & Shimomitsu, T. (2006). Physical activity among the Japanese: Results of the National Health and Nutrition Survey. In *Proceedings of the International Congress on Physical Activity and Public Health April 17–20, 2006* (p. 79). Atlanta, GA: US Department of Health and Human Services.

IPS Correspondents. (2008, 14 August). Paraguay: Concerns, tension rise with water level in Yacyreta Dam. IPS Inter Press Service News Agency. http://www.ipsnews.net/2008/08/paraguay-concerns-tension-rise-with-water-level-in-yacyreta-dam/

Jaacks, L.M., Vandevijvere, S., Pan, A., McGowan, C.J., Wallace, C., Imamura, F., ... & Ezzati, M. (2019). The obesity transition: Stages of the global epidemic. *Lancet Diabetes & Endocrinology, 7*(3), 231–40.

Jaschik, S. (2014, 13 May). The last acceptable prejudice? *Inside Higher Ed.* https://www.insidehighered.com/news/2014/05/13/online-faculty-discussion-raises-concern-about-bias-against-appalachians-and-poor?utm_source=slate&utm_medium=referral&utm_term=partner#sthash.YIbcS7Wf.dpbs

Jordan, B. (1978). *Birth in four cultures: A crosscultural investigation of childbirth in Yucatan, Holland, Sweden, and the United States.* St. Albans, QC: Eden Press.

Jordan, B. (1993). *Birth in four cultures: A crosscultural investigation of childbirth in Yucatan, Holland, Sweden, and the United States* (revised and expanded). Long Grove, IL: Waveland Press.

Jutel, A. (2006). The emergence of overweight as a disease entity: Measuring up normality. *Social Science and Medicine, 63,* 2268–76.

Kahn, M. (1986). *Always hungry, never greedy: Food and the expression of gender in a Melanesian society.* Long Grove, IL: Waveland Press.

Karnehed, N., Rasmussen, F., Hemmingsson, T., & Tynelius, P. (2012). Obesity and attained education: Cohort study of more than 700,000 Swedish men. *Obesity, 14*(8), 1421–8. https://doi.org/10.1038/oby.2006.161

Katare, B., & Beatty, T. (2018). Do environmental factors drive obesity? Evidence from international graduate students. *Health Economics, 27*(10), 1567–93. https://doi-org.ezproxy1.lib.asu.edu/10.1002/hec.3789

Keighley, E., McGarvey, S., Quested, C., McCuddin, C., Viali, S., & Maga, U. (2007). Nutrition and health in modernizing Samoans: Temporal trends and adaptive perspectives. In R. Ohtsuka & S. Ulijaszek (Eds.), *Health change in the Asia–Pacific region* (pp. 147–90). Cambridge, UK: Cambridge University Press.

Klingle, M. (2015). Inescapable paradoxes: Diabetes, progress, and ecologies of inequality. *Environmental History, 20*(4), 736–50. https://doi.org/10.1093/envhis/emv113

Knoema. (2016). *Paraguay – Female obesity prevalence as a share of female ages 18+.* https://knoema.com/atlas/Paraguay/Female-obesity-prevalence

Kondo, D. (1990). *Crafting selves: Power, gender, and discourses of identity in a Japanese workplace.* Chicago, IL: University of Chicago Press.

Krieger, N. (2005). Embodiment: A conceptual glossary for epidemiology. *Journal of Epidemiology & Community Health, 59*(5), 350–5.

Krieger, N. (2016). Living and dying at the crossroads: Racism, embodiment, and why theory is essential for a public health of consequence. *American Journal of Public Health, 106*(5), 832–3. doi: 0.2105/AJPH.2016.303100

Kwan, S. (2009). Individual versus corporate responsibility: Market choice, the food industry, and the pervasiveness of moral models of fatness. *Food, Culture & Society, 12*(4), 477–95.

Lambert, P., & Nickson, A. (2013). *The Paraguay reader: History, culture, politics.* Durham, NC: Duke University Press.

Landecker, H. (2011). Food as exposure: Nutritional epigenetics and the new metabolism. *BioSocieties, 6*(2), 167–94.

Langwick, S.A. (2018). A politics of habitability: Plants, healing, and sovereignty in a toxic world. *Cultural Anthropology, 33*(3), 415–43.

Laymon, K. (2018). *Heavy: An American memoir.* New York, NY: Scribner.

LeBesco, K. (2011). Neoliberalism, public health, and the moral perils of fatness. *Critical Public Health, 21*(2), 153–64.

Lee, J.A., & Pausé, C.J. (2016). Stigma in practice: Barriers to health for fat women. *Frontiers Psychology, 7*(2063), 1–15.

Lester, R. (2019). *Famished: Eating disorders and failed care in America.* Berkeley, CA: University of California Press.

Lilomaiava-Doktor, S. (2009). Beyond "migration": Samoan population movement (Malaga) and the geography of social space (Vā). *The Contemporary Pacific, 21*(1), 1–32.

Livingston, K. (2000). When architecture disables: Teaching undergraduates to perceive ableism in the built environment. *Teaching Sociology, 28*(3), 182–91.

Luhrmann, T.M., Padmavati, R., Tharoor, H., & Osei, A. (2015). Differences in voice-hearing associated with psychosis in Accra, Chennai and San Mateo. *British Journal of Psychiatry, 206*(1), 41–4.

Luke, A., & Cooper, R.S. (2013). Physical activity does not influence obesity risk: Time to clarify the public health message. *International Journal of Epidemiology, 42*(6), 1831–6.

Lunde, F. (2018). *Todo tranquilo: Notions of happiness and well-being in rural and urban Paraguay*. Oslo, Norway: University of Oslo Press.

Lupton, D. (1993). Risk as moral danger: The social and political functions of risk discourse in Public Health. *International Journal of Health Services, 23*(3), 425–35.

Lupton, D. (2012). M-health and health promotion: The digital cyborg and surveillance society. *Social Theory & Health, 10*(3), 229–44.

Lupton, D. (2013). *Fat*. New York, NY: Routledge.

Lutz, C. (1990). The erasure of women's writing in sociocultural anthropology. *American Ethnologist, 17*(4), 611–27.

Macpherson, C., & Macpherson, L. (2010). *The warm winds of change: Globalization in contemporary Samoa*. Auckland, NZ: Auckland University Press.

MacQueen, K., McLellan, E., Kelly, K., & Milstein, B. (1998). Codebook development for team-based qualitative analysis. *Cultural Anthropology Methods, 10*(2), 31–6.

Mah, C. (2010). *Shokuiku*: Governing food and public health in contemporary Japan. *Journal of Sociology, 46*(4), 393–412.

Malinowski, B. (1925). *Coral gardens and their magic: A study of the methods of tilling the soil and of agricultural rites in the Trobriand Islands*. London, UK: Routledge.

Manderson, L. (2016). Anthropological perspectives on the health transition. In S.R. Quah (Ed.), *International Encyclopedia of Public Health* (2nd ed.) (pp. 122–8). Oxford, UK: Academic Press.

Manzenreiter, W. (2012). Monitoring health and the body: Anthropometry, lifestyle risks, and the Japanese obesity crisis. *The Journal of Japanese Studies, 38*(1), 55–84.

Marshall, W.E. (2012). *Potent mana: Lessons in power and healing*. Albany, NY: SUNY Press.

Mauss, M. (1973). Techniques of the body. *Economy and Society, 2*(1), 70–88.

McClure, S. (2013). *"It's Just Gym": Physicality and identity among African American adolescent girls* [Unpublished doctoral dissertation]. Case Western Reserve University.

McCullough, M. (2013). Fat and knocked-up: An embodied analysis of stigma, visibility and invisibility in the biomedical management of an obese pregnancy. In M. McCullough & J. Hardin (Eds.), *Reconstructing obesity research: The measures of meaning, the meaning of measures* (pp. 215–34). New York, NY: Berghahn Books.

McCullough, M., & Hardin, J. (2013). *Reconstructing obesity: The meaning of measures and the measure of meanings*. New York, NY: Berghahn Books.

McGarvey, S. (1992). Economic modernization and human adaptability perspectives. In R. Huss-Ashmore, J. Schall, & M. Hediger (Eds.),

Health and lifestyle change (pp. 105–12). Philadelphia, PA: University of Pennsylvania Museum of Archaeology and Anthropology.

McGarvey, S., & Baker, P.T. (1979). The effects of modernization and migration on Samoan blood pressures. *Human Biology, 51*(4), 461–79.

McLennan, A.K., & Ulijaszek, S. (2015). Obesity emergence in the Pacific Islands: Why understanding colonial history and social change is important. *Public Health Nutrition, 18*(8), 1499–505.

McNaughton, D. (2010). From the womb to the tomb: Obesity and maternal responsibility. *Critical Public Health, 1*, 1–12.

Melby, M., & Takeda, W. (2014). Lifestyle constraints, not inadequate nutrition education, cause gap between breakfast ideals and realities among Japanese in Tokyo. *Appetite, 72*, 37–49. http://dx.doi.org/10.1016/j.appet.2013.09.013

Mendenhall, E. (2016). Beyond comorbidity: A critical perspective of syndemic depression and diabetes in cross-cultural contexts. *Medical Anthropology Quarterly, 30*(4), 462–78. https://doi.org/10.1111/maq.12215

Mendenhall, E. (2019). *Rethinking diabetes: Entanglements with trauma, poverty, and HIV*. Ithaca, NY: Cornell University Press.

Mendenhall, E., Kohrt, B.A., Norris, S.A., Ndetei, D., & Prabhakaran, D. (2017). Non-communicable disease syndemics: Poverty, depression, and diabetes among low-income populations. *Lancet, 389*(10072), 951–63. https://doi.org/10.1016/S0140-6736(17)30402-6

Mihesuah, D.A., & Hoover, E. (2019). *Indigenous food sovereignty in the United States: Restoring cultural knowledge, protecting environments, and regaining health*. Norman, OK: University of Oklahoma Press.

Miller, A. (2016). Asians and obesity: Looks can be deceiving. *US News & World Report*, 11 March. https://health.usnews.com/wellness/articles/2016-03-11/asians-and-obesity-looks-can-be-deceiving

Miller, L. (2006). *Beauty up: Exploring contemporary Japanese body aesthetics*. Berkeley, CA: University of California Press.

Moffat, T. (2010). The "childhood obesity epidemic": Health crisis or social construction? *Medical Anthropology Quarterly, 24*(1), 1–21.

Monaghan, L. (2005). Big handsome men, bears and others: Virtual constructions of "fat male embodiment." *Body & Society, 11*(2), 81–111.

Monaghan, L.F., Colls, R., & Evans, B. (2013). Obesity discourse and fat politics: Research, critique and interventions. *Critical Public Health, 23*(3), 249–62.

Monteiro, C., Moura, E., Conde, W., & Popkin, B. (2004). Socioeconomic status and obesity in adult populations of developing countries: A review. *Bulletin of the World Health Organization, 82*(12), 940–6.

Moran-Thomas, A. (2016). Breakthroughs for whom? Global diabetes care and equitable design. *The New England Journal of Medicine, 375*(24), 2317–19.

Moran-Thomas, A. (2019). What is communicable? Unaccounted injuries and "catching" diabetes in an illegible epidemic. *Cultural Anthropology, 34*(4), 471–502.

Namate, H., Saito, M., & Sawamiya, Y. (2016). Personality traits associated with body shape. *International Journal of Affective Engineering, 15*(2), 161–6.

Narayan, K. (1993). How native is a "native" anthropologist? *American Anthropologist, 95*(3), 671–86.

Navarro, T., Williams, B., & Ahmad, A. (2013). Sitting at the kitchen table: Field notes from women of color in anthropology. *Cultural Anthropology, 28*(3), 443–63.

Nestle, M. (2007). *Food politics: How the food industry influences nutrition and health.* Berkeley, CA: University of California Press.

Nichols, C., Lewis, B.K., & Shreves, M.K. (2015). "Fatties get a room!" An examination of humor and stereotyping in *Mike and Molly. Journal of Entertainment and Media Studies, 1*(1), 99–126.

Nichter, M. (2000). *Fat talk: What girls and their parents say about dieting.* Cambridge, MA: Harvard University Press.

North, S. (2009). *Otoko mo tsurai yo: Dansei no tachiba kara mita shigoto to katei no ryōritsu* [It's tough for men, too: Work–family balance from men's perspective]. In K. Muta (Ed.), *Gendā Sutadīzu* [Gender studies] (pp. 66–88). Osaka, Japan: Osaka University Press.

Ogden, C.L., Carroll, M.D., Fryar, C.D., & Flegal, K.M. (2015). Prevalence of obesity among adults and youth: United States, 2011–2014. *NCHS Data Brief, 219,* November. https://www.cdc.gov/nchs/products/databriefs/db219.html

Ogden, C.L., Carroll, M.D., Kit, B.K., & Flegal, K.M. (2014). Prevalence of childhood and adult obesity in the United States, 2011–2012. *JAMA, 311*(8), 806–14.

Ogden, C.L., Lamb, M.M., Carroll, M.D., & Flegal, K.M. (2010). Obesity and socioeconomic status in adults: United States, 2005–2008. *NCHS Data Brief, 50,* December. https://www.cdc.gov/nchs/data/databriefs/db50.pdf

Ogden, J., Clementi, C., & Aylwin, S. (2006). The impact of obesity surgery and the paradox of control: A qualitative study. *Psychology & Health, 21*(2), 273–93.

Ohnuki-Tierney, E. (1993). *Rice as self: Japanese identities through time.* Princeton, NJ: Princeton University Press.

Oldani, N.O., & Baigún, C.R. (2002). Performance of a fishway system in a major South American dam on the Parana River (Argentina–Paraguay). *River Research and Applications, 18*(2), 171–83.

Omran, A.R. (1971). The epidemiologic transition: A theory of the epidemiology of population change. *The Milbank Memorial Fund Quarterly, 49*(4), 509–38.

Patterson-Faye, C.J. (2016). "I Like the Way You Move": Theorizing fat, Black and sexy. *Sexualities, 19*(8), 926–44.

Phelan, S.M., Burgess, D.J., Yeazel, D.J., Hellerstedt, W.L., Griffin, J.M., & van Ryn, M. (2015). Impact of weight bias and stigma on quality of care and outcomes for patients with obesity. *Obesity Reviews, 16*(4), 319–26. https://doi.org/10.1111/obr.12266

Pike, K., & Borovoy, A. (2004). The rise of eating disorders in Japan: Issues of culture and limitations of the model of "Westernization." *Culture, Medicine and Psychiatry, 28*, 493–531.

Pollock, N. (1992). *These roots remain: Food habits in islands of the Central and Eastern Pacific since Western contact.* Laie, HI: The Institute for Polynesian Studies.

Popenoe, R. (2004). *Feeding desire: Fatness, beauty and sexuality among a Saharan people.* New York, NY: Routledge.

Popkin, B.M. (1994). The nutrition transition in low-income countries: An emerging crisis. *Nutrition Reviews, 52*(9), 285–98.

Popkin, B.M., Adair, L., & Ng, S.W. (2012). Global nutrition transition and the pandemic of obesity in developing countries. *Nutrition Reviews, 70*(1), 3–21.

Popkin, B.M., & Gordon-Larsen, P. (2004). The nutrition transition: Worldwide obesity dynamics and their determinants. *International Journal of Obesity, 28*, 2–9.

Powdermaker, H. (1960). An anthropological approach to the problem of obesity. *Bulletin of the New York Academy of Medicine, 36*(5), 286–95.

Puhl, R., & Brownell, K.D. (2001). Bias, discrimination, and obesity. *Obesity Research, 9*(12), 788–805. https://doi.org/10.1038/oby.2001.108

Puhl, R., & Brownell, K.D. (2006). Confronting and coping with weight stigma: An investigation of overweight and obese adults. *Obesity, 14*(10), 1802–15. https://doi.org/10.1038/oby.2006.208

Puhl, R., & Heuer, C. (2009). The stigma of obesity: A review and update. *Obesity, 17*(5), 941–64. https://doi.org/10.1038/oby.2008.636

Puhl, R., & Heuer, C. (2010). Obesity stigma: Important considerations for public health. *American Journal of Public Health, 100*(6), 1019–28.

Puhl, R., Peterson, J.L., & Luedicke, J. (2013). Fighting obesity or obese persons? Public perceptions of obesity-related health messages. *International Journal of Obesity, 37*(6), 774–82. https://doi.org/10.1038/ijo.2012.156

Raskin, S.E. (2015). *Decayed, missing, and filled: Subjectivity and the dental safety net in central Appalachia* [Unpublished doctoral dissertation]. University of Arizona.

Raskin, S.E. (2017). "Toothless maw-maw can't eat no more": Stigma and synergies of dental disease, diabetes, and psychosocial stress among low-income rural Appalachians. In B. Ostrach, S. Lerman, & M. Singer (Eds.), *Stigma syndemics: New directions in biosocial health* (pp. 193–216). Lanham, MD: Lexington Books.

Reese, A. (2018). "We will not perish; we're going to keep flourishing": Race, food access, and geographies of self-reliance. *Antipode, 50*(2), 407–24.

Reese, A. (2019). *Black food geographies: Race, self-reliance, and food access in Washington.* Chapel Hill, NC: UNC Press Books.

Reiter, R., & Rapp, R. (Eds.). (1975). *Toward an anthropology of women.* New York, NY: Monthly Review Press.

Roberts, E. (2015). Food is love: And so, what then? *BioSocieties, 10,* 247–52. doi:10.1057/biosoc.2015.18.

Roberts, E. (2017). What gets inside: Violent entanglements and toxic boundaries in Mexico City. *Cultural Anthropology, 32*(4), 592–619.

Rogge, M.M. (2004). Obesity, stigma, and civilized oppression. *Advances in Nursing Science, 27*(4), 301–15.

Romero, S. (2012). An indigenous language with unique staying power. *The New York Times,* 12 March. http://www.nytimes.com/2012/03/12/world/americas/in-paraguay-indigenous-language-with-unique-staying-power.html.

Rosaldo, M., & Lamphere, L. (1974). *Woman, culture, and society.* Stanford, CA: Stanford University Press.

Rose, N. (2006). *The politics of life itself: Biomedicine, power, and subjectivity in the twenty-first century.* Princeton, NJ: Princeton University Press.

Rose, N., & Novas, C. (2007). Biological citizenship. In A. Ong & S.J. Collier (Eds.), *Global assemblages: Technology, politics, and ethics as anthropological problems* (pp. 439–63). Oxford, UK: Blackwell Publishing.

Rothblum, E., & Solovay, S. (2009). *The fat studies reader.* New York, NY: New York University Press.

Rubin, L.R., Fitts, M.L., & Becker, A.E. (2003). "Whatever feels good in my soul": Body ethics and aesthetics among African American and Latina women. *Culture, Medicine & Psychiatry, 27*(1), 49–75.

Saguy, A.C. (2012). Why fat is a feminist issue. *Sex Roles, 66,* 600–7.

Saguy, A.C. (2013). *What's wrong with fat?* London, UK: Oxford University Press.

Saguy, A.C., & Almeling, R. (2008). Fat in the fire? Science, the news media, and the "obesity epidemic." *Sociological Review, 23*(1), 53–83.

Saguy, A.C., & Riley, K. (2005). Weighing both sides: Morality, mortality, and framing contests over obesity. *Journal of Health Politics, 30*(5), 869–921.

Saguy, A.C., & Ward, A. (2011). Coming out as fat: Rethinking stigma. *Social Psychology Quarterly, 74*(1), 53–75. https://doi.org/10.1177/0190272511398190

Salant, T., & Santry, H.P. (2006). Internet marketing of bariatric surgery: Contemporary trends in the medicalization of society. *Social Science & Medicine, 62,* 2445–57.

Saldaña-Tejeda, A. (2017). Mitochondrial mothers of a fat nation: Race, gender and epigenetics in obesity research on Mexican Mestizos. *BioSocieties, 13*(2), 434–52.

Saldaña-Tejeda, A., & Wade, P. (2018). Obesity, race and the indigenous origins of health risks among Mexican mestizos. *Ethnic and Racial Studies, 41*(15), 2731–49. https://doi.org/10.1080/01419870.2017.1407810

Saldaña-Tejeda, A., & Wade, P. (2019). Eugenics, epigenetics, and obesity predisposition among Mexican Mestizos. *Medical Anthropology, 38*(8), 664–79.

Samoan Bureau of Statistics. (2011). *Population and housing census 2011.* Global Health Data Exchange. http://ghdx.healthdata.org/record/samoa-population-and-housing-census-2011

Sanabria, E. (2016). Circulating ignorance: Complexity and agnogenesis in the obesity "epidemic." *Cultural Anthropology, 31*(1), 131–58. https://doi.org/10.14506/ca31.1.07

Sanabria, E., & Yates-Doerr, E. (2015). Alimentary uncertainties: From contested evidence to policy. *BioSocieties, 10*(2), 117–24.

Scheper-Hughes, N., & Lock, N. (1987). The mindful body: A prolegomenon to future work in medical anthropology. *Medical Anthropology Quarterly, 1*(1), 6–41.

Schnegg, M., & Lowe, E.D. (Eds.). (2020). *Comparing cultures: Innovations in comparative ethnography.* New York, NY: Cambridge University Press.

Schwartz, M.B., Chambliss, H.O., Brownell, K.D., Blair, S.N., & Billington, C. (2003). Weight bias among health professionals specializing in obesity. *Obesity Research, 11*(9), 1033–9. https://doi.org/10.1038/oby.2003.142

Seversen, A. (2019). Why I'm trading body positivity for fat acceptance. *Healthline,* 13 June. https://www.healthline.com/health/fat-acceptance-vs-body-positivity#1

Shafer, B.E. (Ed.). (1991). *Is America different? A new look at American exceptionalism.* Oxford, UK: Oxford University Press.

Singer, M. (2014). Following the turkey tails: Neoliberal globalization and the political ecology of health. *Journal of Political Ecology, 21*(1), 437–51.

Smith, L.T. (1999). *Decolonizing methodologies: Research and Indigenous peoples.* London, UK: Zed Books.

Snowdon, W., & Thow, A.M. (2013). Trade policy and obesity prevention: Challenges and innovation in the Pacific Islands. *Obesity Reviews 14*(52), 150–8.

Sobo, E.J. (1994). The sweetness of fat: Health, procreation, and sociability in rural Jamaica. In N. Sault (Ed.), *Many mirrors: Body image and social relations* (pp. 133–53). New Brunswick, NJ: Rutgers University Press.

Solomon, H. (2015, 20 April). Fat: Deviation. *Society for Cultural Anthropology.* https://culanth.org/fieldsights/fat-deviation

Solomon, H. (2016). *Metabolic living: Food, fat, and the absorption of illness in India.* Durham, NC: Duke University Press.

State of Childhood Obesity. (n.d.). Georgia. Accessed 9 December 2020. https://stateofobesity.org/states/ga

Stearns, P. (2002). *Fat history: Bodies and beauty in the modern west.* New York, NY: New York University Press.

Strings, S. (2019). Fearing the Black body: The racial origins of fat phobia. New York, NY: New York University Press.

SturtzSreetharan, C. (2004). Students, *sarariiman* (pl.), and seniors: Japanese men's use of "manly" speech register. *Language in Society, 33*, 81–107.

SturtzSreetharan, C. (2006). Gentlemanly gender? Japanese men's politeness in casual conversations. *Journal of Sociolinguistics, 10*(1), 70–92.

SturtzSreetharan, C. (2009). *"Ore" and "omae"*: Japanese men's use of first- and second-person pronouns. *Pragmatics, 19*(2), 253–78.

SturtzSreetharan, C. (2017). Language and masculinity: The role of Osaka dialect in contemporary ideals of fatherhood. *Gender & Language, 11*(4), 552–74.

SturtzSreetharan, C., Agostini, G., Brewis, A., & Wutich, A. (2019). Fat talk: A citizen sociolinguistic approach. *Journal of Sociolinguistics, 23*(3), 263–83.

SturtzSreetharan, C., & Brewis, A. (2019). Rice, men, and other everyday anxieties: Navigating obesogenic urban food environments in Osaka, Japan. In I. Vojnovic, A. Pearson, A. Gershim, G. Deverteuil, & A. Allen (Eds.), *Handbook of global urban health* (pp. 545–64). New York, NY: Routledge.

SturtzSreetharan, C., Trainer, S., Wutich, A., & Brewis, A. (2018). Moral biocitizenship: Discursively managing food and the body after bariatric surgery. *Journal of Linguistic Anthropology, 28*(2), 221–40.

Takeda, H. (2008). Delicious food in a beautiful country: Nationhood and nationalism in discourses on food in contemporary Japan. *Studies in Ethnicity and Nationalism, 8*(1), 5–30.

Takeda, W., & Melby, M.K. (2017). Spatial, temporal, and health associations of eating alone: A cross-cultural analysis of young adults in urban Australia and Japan. *Appetite, 118*, 149–60.

Takeda, W., Melby, M.K., & Ishikawa, Y. (2017). Food education for whom? Perceptions of food education and literacy among dietitians and laypeople in urban Japan. *Food Studies: An Interdisciplinary Journal, 7*(4), 49–66.

Takeda, W., Melby, M.K., & Ishikawa, Y. (2018). Who eats with family and how often? Household members and work styles influence frequency of family meals in urban Japan. *Appetite, 125*, 160–71.

Tanaka, N., & Kinoshita, Y. (2009). The importance of nutritional education in preventing obesity and malnutrition. *Forum on Public Policy Online, 2009*(1). https://eric.ed.gov/?id=EJ864752

Tanaka, S., Itō, Y., & Hattori, K. (2002). Relationship of body composition to body-fatness estimation in Japanese university students. *Obesity Research, 10*(7), 590–6.

Taylor, N. (2011). Negotiating popular obesity discourses in adolescence. *Food, Culture & Society, 14*(4), 587–606. https://doi.org/10.2752/175174411X13046092851433

Taylor, N. (2015). *Schooled on fat: What teens tell us about gender, body image, and obesity.* New York, NY: Routledge.

Thompson, C. (2017, 4 May). Fat-positive activists explain what it's really like to be fat. *Vice.* https://www.vice.com/en_us/article/gvzx94/fat-positive-activists-explain-what-its-really-like-to-be-fat

Tomiyama, A.J., Carr, D., Granberg, E.M., Major, B., Robinson, E., Sutin, A.R., & Brewis, A. (2018). How and why weight stigma drives the obesity "epidemic" and harms health. *BMC Medicine, 16*(123). https://doi.org/10.1186/s12916-018-1116-5

Tovar, V. (2019, 18 September). *Virgie Tovar tells us the difference between body positivity and fat activism.* [Video]. YouTube. https://www.youtube.com/watch?v=o_OoS_hgXfQ

Tracy, S. (2010). Qualitative quality: Eight "big-tent" criteria for excellent qualitative research. *Field Methods, 16*(10), 837–51.

Trainer, S. (2013). Body image and weight concerns among Emirati women in the United Arab Emirates. In M. McCullough & J. Hardin (Eds.), *Reconstructing obesity: The meaning of measures and the measure of meaning* (pp. 147–68). New York, NY: Berghahn Books.

Trainer, S. (2017). Glocalizing beauty: Weight and body image in the new Middle East. In E. Anderson-Fye & A. Brewis (Eds.), *Fat planet: Obesity, culture, and symbolic capital* (pp. 171–92). Sante Fe, NM: University of New Mexico Press.

Trainer, S., Brewis, A., Hruschka, D., & Williams, D. (2015). Translating obesity: Navigating the front lines of the "war on fat." *American Journal of Human Biology, 27*(1), 61–8. https://doi.org/10.1002/ajhb.22623

Trainer, S., Brewis, A., Williams, D., & Chavez, J.R. (2015). Obese, fat, or "just big"? Young adult deployment of and reactions to weight terms. *Human Organization, 74*(3), 266–75. https://doi.org/10.17730/0018-7259-74.3.266

Trainer, S., Brewis, A., & Wutich, A. (2017). Not "taking the easy way out": Reframing bariatric surgery from low-effort weight loss to hard work. *Anthropology & Medicine, 24*(1), 96–110.

Trainer, S., Brewis, A., & Wutich, A. (2020). *Extreme weight loss: Struggling with weight before and after bariatric surgery.* New York, NY: New York University Press.

Trainer, S., Brewis, A., Wutich, A., Kurtz, L., & Niesluchowski, M. (2016). The fat self in virtual communities: Success and failure in weight-loss blogging. *Current Anthropology, 57*(4), 523–8.

Trainer, S., Hardin, J., SturtzSreetharan, C., & Brewis, A. (2020). Worry-nostalgia: Anxieties around the felt fading of local cuisines and foodways. *Gastronomica*, Summer, 67–78.

Trainer, S., Wutich, A., & Brewis, A. (2017). Eating in the panopticon: Surveillance of food and weight before and after bariatric surgery. *Medical Anthropology, 36*(5), 500–14. https://doi.org/10.1080/01459740.2017.1298595

Traphagan, J., & Brown, K. (2002). Fast food and intergenerational commensality in Japan: New styles and old patters. *Ethnology, 41*(2), 119–34.

Trnka, S., & Trundle, C. (Eds.). (2017). *Competing responsibilities: The ethics and politics of contemporary life.* Durham, NC: Duke University Press Books.

Turner, B.S. (1982). The discourse of diet. *Theory, Culture & Society, 1*(1): 23–32.

Turner, B.S. (1984). *The body and society: Explorations in social theory.* Thousand Oaks, CA: Sage.

Ultima Hora. (2011, 17 August). El 50 % de la población paraguaya tiene sobrepeso. http://www.ultimahora.com/el-50-la-poblacion-paraguaya-tiene-sobrepeso-n455243.html

Unnithan-Kumar, M., & Tremayne, S. (2011). *Fatness and the maternal body: Women's experiences of corporeality and the shaping of social policy.* New York, NY: Berghahn Books.

Valdez, N. (2018). The redistribution of reproductive responsibility: On the epigenetics of "environment" in prenatal interventions. *Medical Anthropology Quarterly, 32*(3), 425–42.

Vogel, E., & Mol, A. (2014). Enjoy your food: On losing weight and taking pleasure. *Sociology of Health and Illness, 36*(2), 305–17.

Wakita, H. (1999). Ports, markets, and medieval urbanism in the Osaka region. In J. McClain & O. Wakita (Eds.), *Osaka: The merchants' capital of early modern Japan* (pp. 22–44). Ithaca, NY: Cornell University Press.

Warin, M. (2009). *Abject relations: Everyday worlds of anorexia.* New Brunswick, NJ: Rutgers University Press.

Warin, M., & Gunson, J. (2013). The weight of the word: Knowing silences in obesity research. *Qualitative Health Research, 23*(12), 1686–96.

Warin, M., Moore, V., Davies, M., & Ulijaszek, S. (2016). Epigenetics and obesity: The reproduction of habitus through intracellular and social environments. *Body & Society, 22*(4), 53–78.

Warin, M., Moore, V., Zivkovic, T., & Davies, M. (2011). Telescoping the origins of obesity to women's bodies: How gender inequalities are being squeezed out of Barker's Hypothesis. *Annals of Human Biology, 38*(4), 453–60.

Warin, M., Turner, K., Moore, V., & Davies, M. (2008). Bodies, mothers and identities: Rethinking obesity and the BMI. *Sociology of Health & Illness, 30*(1), 97–111.

Warin, M., & Zivkovic, T. (2019). *Fatness, obesity, and disadvantage in the Australian suburbs: Unpalatable politics.* New York, NY: Palgrave Macmillan.

Warin, M., Zivkovic, T., Moore, V., & Davies, M. (2012). Mothers as smoking guns: Fetal overnutrition and the reproduction of obesity. *Feminism & Psychology, 22*(3), 360–75.

Watkins, P.L. (2015). Fat studies 101: Learning to have your cake and eat it too. *M/C Journal, 18*(3). http://journal.media-culture.org.au/index.php/mcjournal/article/view/968

Watkins, P.L., Farrell, A., & Hugmeyer, A.D. (2012). Teaching fat studies: From conception to reception. *Fat Studies, 1*(2), 180–94. https://doi.org/10.1080/21604851.2012.649232

Weaver, L.J. (2018). *Sugar and tension: Diabetes and gender in modern India.* New Brunswick, NJ: Rutgers University Press.

Weber, M. (2002). *The Protestant ethic and the "spirit" of capitalism and other writings* (P. Baehr & G.C. Wells, Trans.). New York, NY: Penguin Books.

Weiner, A. (1976). *Women of value, men of renown: New perspectives in Trobriand Exchange.* Austin, TX: University of Texas Press.

Welch, W. (Ed.). (2014). *Public health in Appalachia: Essays from the clinic and the field.* Jefferson, NC: McFarland and Co.

Whiting, B. (Ed.). (1963). *Six cultures: Studies in child rearing.* New York, NY: John Wiley & Sons.

Wiedman, D. (2012). Native American embodiment of the chronicities of modernity: Reservation food, diabetes, and the metabolic syndrome among the Kiowa, Comanche, and Apache. *Medical Anthropology Quarterly, 26*(4), 95–612.

Wolf, D. (1996). *Feminist dilemmas in fieldwork.* Boulder, CO: Westview Press.

Wolfe, A. (2017a, 25 September). Eating in the Delta: A community uses soil to fight food insecurity, promote sovereignty. *The Clarion Ledger.* http:// www.clarionledger.com/story/news/politics/2017/09/25/hunger -food-desert-mississippi-delta-community/685223001/

Wolfe, A. (2017b, 24 September). Surrounded by crops, lacking food: A health paradox in the Mississippi Delta. *The Clarion Ledger.* http://www .clarionledger.com/story/news/politics/2017/09/24/hunger-food -desert-mississippi-delta-impacts-health/588052001/

World Health Organization. (2004). Appropriate body-mass index for Asian populations and its implications for policy and intervention strategies. *Lancet, 363,* 157–63. https://www.who.int/nutrition/publications/bmi _asia_strategies.pdf

World Health Organization. (2016). Paraguay. Diabetes country profiles. http://www.who.int/diabetes/country-profiles/pry_en.pdf

Wray, S., & Deery, R. (2008). The medicalization of body size and women's health care. *Health Care for Women International, 29*(3), 227–43. https:// doi.org/10.1080/07399330701738291

Wutich, A., & Brewis, A. (2019). Data collection in cross-cultural ethnographic studies. *Field Methods, 31*(2), 181–9.

Wutich, A., Roberts, C., White, D., Larson, K., & Brewis, A. (2014). Hard paths, soft paths, or no paths? Cross cultural perceptions of water solutions. *Hydrology & Earth Systems Science, 18,* 109–20.

Yates-Doerr, E. (2012). The weight of the self: Care and compassion in Guatemalan dietary choices. *Medical Anthropology Quarterly, 26*(1), 136–58. https://doi.org/10.1111/j.1548-1387.2011.01169.x

Yates-Doerr, E. (2014). The mismeasure of obesity. In M. McCullough & J. Hardin (Eds.), *Reconstructing obesity research: The measures of meaning, the meaning of measures* (pp. 49–70). New York, NY: Berghahn Books.

Yates-Doerr, E. (2015). *The weight of obesity: Hunger and global health in postwar Guatemala.* Berkeley, CA: University of California Press.

Yates-Doerr, E. (2020). Antihero Care: On fieldwork and anthropology. *Anthropology & Humanism 45*(2): 233–44. https://doi.org/10.1111/anhu.12300

Young, M.W. (1972). *Fighting with food: Leadership, values and social control in a Massim society.* New York, NY: Cambridge University Press.

Zigon, J. (2008). *Morality: An anthropological perspective.* Oxford, UK: Bloomsbury Press.

Zivkovic, T., Warin, M., Davies, M., & Moore, V. (2010). In the name of the child: The gendered politics of childhood obesity. *Journal of Sociology, 46*(4), 375–92.

Index

Page numbers in italics represent photos/figures, *t* represents tables.

⏵ TEACHING CULTURE
Ethnographies for the Classroom

Editor: John Barker, University of British Columbia

This series is an essential resource for instructors searching for ethnographic case studies that are contemporary, engaging, provocative, and created specifically with undergraduate students in mind. Written with clarity and personal warmth, books in the series introduce students to the core methods and orienting frameworks of ethnographic research and provide a compelling entry point to some of the most urgent issues faced by people around the globe today.

Recent Books in the Series

Fat in Four Cultures: A Global Ethnography of Weight by Cindi SturtzSreetharan, Alexandra Brewis, Jessica Hardin, Sarah Trainer, and Amber Wutich (2021)

Esperanza Speaks: Confronting a Century of Global Change in Rural Panama by Gloria Rudolf (2021)

The Living Inca Town: Tourist Encounters in the Peruvian Andes by Karoline Guelke (2021)

Collective Care: Indigenous Motherhood, Family, and HIV/AIDS by Pamela J. Downe (2021)

I Was Never Alone, or Oporniki: An Ethnographic Play on Disability in Russia by Cassandra Hartblay (2020)

Millennial Movements: Positive Social Change in Urban Costa Rica by Karen Stocker (2020)

From Water to Wine: Becoming Middle Class in Angola by Jess Auerbach (2020)

Deeply Rooted in the Present: Heritage, Memory, and Identity in Brazilian Quilombos by Mary Lorena Kenny (2018)

Long Night at the Vepsian Museum: The Forest Folk of Northern Russia and the Struggle for Cultural Survival by Veronica Davidov (2017)

Truth and Indignation: Canada's Truth and Reconciliation Commission on Indian Residential Schools, second edition, by Ronald Niezen (2017)

Merchants in the City of Art: Work, Identity, and Change in a Florentine Neighborhood by Anne Schiller (2016)

Ancestral Lines: The Maisin of Papua New Guinea and the Fate of the Rainforest, second edition, by John Barker (2016)

Love Stories: Language, Private Love, and Public Romance in Georgia by
  Paul Manning (2015)
Culturing Bioscience: A Case Study in the Anthropology of Science by
  Udo Krautwurst (2014)
Fields of Play: An Ethnography of Children's Sports by Noel Dyck (2012)
Made in Madagascar: Sapphires, Ecotourism, and the Global Bazaar by
  Andrew Walsh (2012)
Red Flags and Lace Coiffes: Identity and Survival in a Breton Village by
  Charles R. Menzies (2011)
*Rites of the Republic: Citizens' Theatre and the Politics of Culture in
  Southern France* by Mark Ingram (2011)